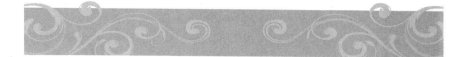

Heal Your Skin

THE BREAKTHROUGH PLAN
FOR RENEWAL

Ava Shamban, M.D.

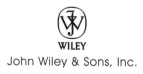

WILEY

John Wiley & Sons, Inc.

To Nancy Daly, who worked tirelessly on behalf of foster youth,
music, and the fine arts, never faltering in the face of serious illness

To Zack, Reid, and Dylan, who inspire me with their
endless curiosity and pursuit of their personal best

And to my parents, who encouraged me to challenge myself
and always emphasized the importance of giving back

This book is printed on acid-free paper. ♾

Copyright © 2011 by Ava Shamban, M.D.
   All rights reserved

All artwork by BMKT.

Published by John Wiley & Sons, Inc., Hoboken,
   New Jersey
Published simultaneously in Canada

Design and composition by Forty-five Degree
   Design LLC

The information contained in this book is not intended to serve as a replacement for professional medical advice. Any use of the information in this book is at the reader's discretion. The author and the publisher specifically disclaim any and all liability arising directly or indirectly from the use or application of any information contained in this book. A health care professional should be consulted regarding your specific situation.

For general information about our other products and services, please contact our Customer Care Department within the United States at (800) 762-2974, outside the United States at (317) 572-3993 or fax (317) 572-4002.

Wiley also publishes its books in a variety of electronic formats. Some content that appears in print may not be available in electronic books. For more information about Wiley products, visit our web site at www.wiley.com.

ISBN 978-0470-53215-7 (paper)
ISBN 978-1118-01963-4 (ebk)
ISBN 978-1118-01964-1 (ebk)
ISBN 978-1118-01965-8 (ebk)

Printed in the United States of America

10 9 8 7 6 5 4 3 2 1

CONTENTS

ACKNOWLEDGMENTS

If it takes a village to raise a child, it certainly takes a metropolis to write a book. The large community of my metropolis who have encouraged and supported me, exhorted and stimulated me includes many to whom I owe thanks and gratitude:

First and foremost are my patients, who have taught me more than I could ever learn from any book, and my office staff, always supportive and understanding.

My professors at Harvard University and my initial research experience at the Seymour Kety lab at McLean Hospital have been instrumental in my career. The outstanding medical education and training that I received at Case Western Reserve Medical School and UCLA–Harbor Medical Center was invaluable, as was my fellowship year with my mentor and friend, Jouni Uitto, M.D., Ph.D.

It would take another book to list everything I've learned from my companion physicians and the production team at *Extreme Makeover*, and now my new colleagues at *The Doctors*: Carla Pennington, Michelle Wendt, and Andrew Scher, who work hard every day trying to make medicine more accessible and easier to understand. Clearly, *Heal Your Skin* has been influenced by those noble goals.

I am indebted to my colleagues Dr. Vic Narukar, Dr. Ken Beer, Dr. George Martin, and Dr. Susan Weinkle, who provide me with opportunities to collaborate on many projects as well as advance the field of dermatology.

An endless supply of thank-yous to all my friends who kept telling me I could write a book, until finally, even I believed them. Especially Holly Hein, who has consistently supported me through the ups and downs of life, family, and work.

The earlier stages of this book were brought to life with assistance from Julie Logan and Tim Green. As the process continued, Holly Goldberg Sloan, Natasha Singer, Judith Newman, Joanne McPortland, and Judy Freed made important contributions. Thank you to my amazing agent, Loretta Barrett, and attorney, Susan Grode, and to the incredible team at John Wiley & Sons. They believed in this book from the very beginning.

A very special thanks and deepest gratitude is given to my friend Kathy Ann Stumpe. Her expertise, sense of humor, deep emotional investment, and willingness to sit for hours with me as we wrote allowed the book to come to life in a form that speaks to all.

Finally, I'd like to acknowledge Isabella Toma, who worked extensively on this book from the start. She always understood how important it was for me to write *Heal Your Skin*, and she helped make it happen.

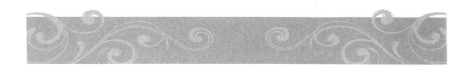

Introduction

I am a healer. It's what I've always wanted to be, even as a child. When my friends were busy reading books about girl detectives, I was reading books about science, medicine, and the life of the celebrated English nurse Florence Nightingale.

My interest in the skin did not begin in earnest until after I finished my basic training as a physician and became a general practitioner, serving migrant farmworkers in central California. My practice covered everything from prenatal care to geriatrics. Many of my patients suffered inordinately from skin conditions. They came to see me with acne or allergic reactions to the plants they were handling in the fields. At the time, I simply did not have the necessary skills to treat them. I referred them to dermatologists in the community, but there were very few of these doctors available. Sometimes my patients had to wait up to three months to see a skin specialist.

I began to study the skin in more depth. This led me to have a much greater understanding not only of this organ's marvelous and intricate scientific workings but also of how the condition of our skin affects our lives at the most basic level. Our skin reflects our body's inner state of health, but the skin's own health and well-being also have a major impact on our self-esteem and our quality of life, as study after study has shown.

Under a fellowship program, I examined the molecular underpinnings of inherited skin diseases that involve two major proteins, collagen and elastin. I completed my residency at Harbor-UCLA Hospital, where I treated patients with an enormous range of skin conditions. This residency also gave me a greater appreciation for the basic beauty of the skin in all its types and ethnicities. Polynesians, Asians, African Americans, Latinos, and Caucasians: it was truly a melting pot of skin experiences.

It has been said that in life, timing is everything. This was certainly true for me, because the end of my residency coincided with the introduction of lasers and other forms of nonsurgical interventions for skin issues and problems. Science was helping us to do more and more to treat what had been untreatable in the past. It was a fascinating blend of science and aesthetics. I began attending numerous conferences and training seminars, learning how to use lasers to treat birthmarks, eliminate wrinkles, and remove brown spots.

In the beginning, there were only three types of lasers at our disposal. Now there are more than two hundred. The challenge for me was to learn how to use this new technology in combination with traditional skin care to rejuvenate a face or to repair an area of the body that had been damaged by trauma, such as a car accident or a dog bite. One of my most memorable cases involved a woman whose parrot bit her lip!

I became known as a laser specialist in Los Angeles. I also started to use injectables to add volume to the face, giving it a more beautiful look rather than the stretched-tight face that had been the only "rejuvenation" option in the past.

Then, I was asked to be the dermatologist for the reality show *Extreme Makeover*. The dermatology work on the program ranged from treating acne scars to rejuvenating the skin of a woman with breast cancer. During my work on the show, I had to learn how to achieve results in a short amount of time instead of the three to six months that is usually required in dermatology. Furthermore, I had to get those results in front of eight million viewers. It was a daunting professional challenge, to say the least.

I knew I'd have to call on all the tools and knowledge I'd acquired from working in every aspect of medicine in my career, including lab research, clinical research, medical dermatology, and aesthetic dermatology. I discovered that by using different combinations of lasers, anti-inflammatories, and other skin treatments, I could get the desired results in the required time frame.

Next to having my children, this was the most profound experience of my life, because I had the privilege of watching the lives of these people being transformed, along with their appearance. As a physician, I may see the same patient once a month or perhaps every other week. Because I saw the *Extreme Makeover* patients two or three times a week, I really began to understand what transforming their skin meant to them. A lot of us are blessed with reasonably good looks and enjoy good health. We cannot comprehend how tormented a person can be just by looking in a mirror and seeing terribly unhealthy skin. We fail to realize how liberating it can be to see our reflection and say three simple words: "I look great."

The *Extreme Makeover* patients evolved from their participation in the show, and so did I. I became a better doctor. On a deeper level, I became a better healer because I understood the impact this work could have. It was inspiring. In fact, it inspired me to write this book.

How many of us have had a stressful workweek or a personal relationship problem and then found our skin breaking out, as in our teenage years, though we thought that skin problem had been solved? How many of us wander through the uncharted territory of menopause, wondering why our skin flares red, turns white, and then suddenly gets brown spots—all while turning as dry as the Sahara? I have realized that there are many different populations of people who go from doctor to doctor, unable to get their skin care goals or needs met.

People have told me over and over that they want their skin to look and feel great, no matter what else is going on in their lives. This book has one goal: to provide you with a simple source of information on both common and uncommon skin issues. There are hundreds of books about skin care, and I've read most of them. Some are more useful than others. So before I even typed the first word, I knew that this book would have to accomplish three key goals:

It has to provide proven solutions to skin care problems. I don't mean solutions that require you to see a dermatologist. Of course, it is sometimes necessary to get help from a health care provider. For the most part, however, all of my skin care plans are designed to show you what you can do now, at home, to heal your skin and to look and feel amazing. My practice has treated more than fifty thousand patients, and many of the solutions I reveal in this book come directly from them. We know what works—and what doesn't—and now you get to benefit from all that experience. I've even included case studies from my patient files to explain different skin challenges and how we treated them.

It has to be easy to understand. A few years ago, I bought a camera but found the manual so confusing that the camera sat in my drawer for months before I ever took one photo. When I wrote this book, I wanted to present medical knowledge and scientific background in a way that would be understandable, approachable, and, most of all, usable.

It has to provide expert advice. I assembled a team of experts to provide me with their most current knowledge on how skin is affected by acne, pregnancy, menopause, and serious illnesses, including cancer, and on the role that nutrition and fitness play in our ongoing skin health. This team included Dr. Dianne Rosenberg, a specialist in obstetrics and gynecology; Dr. Wendy Bazilian, a doctor of public health and a registered dietitian; and Alisa Daglio, a fitness trainer who worked with me on *Extreme Makeover*.

I know how stressful it can be when your skin is not looking or feeling its best. It can affect every part of your life. Even more stressful is not knowing what you can do right now to care for your skin. As a doctor and a healer, my job is to show you how you can take your skin from troubled to terrific. It's as easy as turning the page.

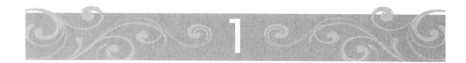

Life Happens, but It Doesn't Have to Show on Your Skin

s your life showing on your skin—and you're panicked?

Maybe it is, if any of these scenarios sounds familiar:

- The stress from your job, your family, or both is making you break out more than you ever did as a teenager.
- You're thrilled to be pregnant, but you look at your expanding belly and discover there are angry red stripes and even a dark line right down the middle that make the idea of ever wearing a bikini again just terrifying.
- You pull out a compact to check if your latest hot flash has melted your mascara, and you notice a wrinkle that you swear wasn't there the day before.

As a board-certified dermatologist in practice for more than twenty years, I've treated thousands of patients whose skin has been under assault from stress, aging, and illness. Through a careful process of treatments designed to heal the skin, I have learned this lesson: Life happens, but it doesn't have to show on your skin.

Patients come to me because their skin problems have left them feeling frustrated and helpless. They don't know what to do or where to turn for answers, and they're unhappy with the poor image they're showing the world. Healthy skin is like a smile on your face; it projects a state of well-being, happiness, and peace.

Since some of my patients are celebrities, I'm sometimes known as the Red Carpet Dermatologist. However, I understand that whether you're going to the Oscars, the office, or your local grocery store, you still want your skin to look great. And no, it's not a matter of vanity. Studies have shown a direct correlation between appearance and quality of life. People who feel good about their appearance usually feel good about life in general.

I know the frustration and helplessness that accompany serious skin challenges. That's what brings patients to my practice every day, seeking real solutions. When your skin is under assault—from stress-related acne outbreaks, the turmoil of hormonal changes, or the collateral damage that skin suffers from other causes—your whole life is affected. The surface of your skin both expresses and influences what's happening in the rest of your life. It also reflects what's happening inside your body. This is a connection that many of us fail to take into account when we try to heal our skin. That is why I always try to place my patients' skin problems in the context of any other health issues in order to give them the best result from my care.

Even though many of my patients are in the public eye, I can tell you that we're all the same when our skin is under assault. We want answers. We want help—and we want it now.

That's why I'm here. There *are* answers. You aren't helpless, and improving your life by healing your skin is no idle hope. It's a reality that started the minute you picked up this book.

Going to Extremes

As a dermatologist, my goal is to heal my patients' skin in order to help them achieve a positive change in their lives. My scientific training began at Harvard University and continued in the laboratory, where I investigated the expression of the collagen and elastin genes. Through this intensive learning process, I came to understand how skin works, so I am able to give my patients the benefit of my basic science background. When I joined the team of professionals on ABC television's *Extreme Makeover*, I brought the skill of skin healing to the team.

As initially conceived, the show's Extreme Team didn't include a dermatologist. As a result, both the subjects and the professionals noticed that something was missing. If the skin isn't healthy, a physical transformation isn't complete. Healthy, renewed skin is the gift wrap on the makeover. I participated in the show for a trial run, and my work with the team was an alchemy so successful that I stayed with the show for its duration.

From working with the participants on the show, I learned how to implement a combination approach that employs every tool at my disposal (lasers, peels, and an at-home regimen) to get the best possible results in the fastest time possible. My goal now is to have you benefit from my experience and my unique approach to healing your skin.

Outside In

Let me be very clear: we're not talking about vanity. Healthy, beautiful skin is high on the list of your personal bill of rights. We are all entitled to it. If your skin and your spirit are already under assault, your desire for better skin should be encouraged.

"You don't have acne, you're just vain," a general practitioner once told one of my patients, a high-powered executive in her forties who knew very well that she was losing confidence (and her edge in a competitive industry) with every disfiguring flare. Doctors often tell women that they're being silly to seek solutions for pregnancy- or menopause-related skin changes. The often life-limiting side effects of serious illness on the skin can be overlooked. "How you look or feel right now doesn't matter," patients often hear. "Let's save your life now and worry about your skin later."

Yet if those patients feel good about their appearance, they heal faster, cooperate more energetically with treatment, and sustain positive outcomes longer. If they feel bad about their appearance, this can actually slow down healing, cooperation, and positive outcomes. Dr. Robert Klitzman, a professor of clinical psychiatry at Columbia University Medical Center, has noted, "Aesthetic assaults on patients can contribute to depression and anxiety that could in turn hamper patients in treating and caring for themselves. . . . We are not only biological creatures but social, symbolic, and aesthetic ones as well. We ignore any one of these attributes only at a cost."

The Skills for Healing

If you are unhappy about how your skin looks, you don't have to waste any more time. I have written this book to provide information and solutions for every skin type and for some of the most difficult challenges your skin can face, such as persistent or adult-onset acne, hormonal changes, the effects of aging, or the effects of serious illness. This book is for you if you're dealing with any of these challenges, if you care about someone who is, or if you just want to know what could happen. (Statistically speaking, you are likely to face at least one of them.) In the pages ahead, we will cover each challenge specifically so you will learn the following:

- What is going on with your skin
- How to heal it
- How to maintain great-looking skin

We will also talk about the science of the skin and the basics of everyday skin care. Because I know that the state of your skin reflects how well you are eating and taking care of your body, I've asked celebrity nutritionist Dr. Wendy Bazilian and fitness coach Alisa Daglio (another member of the Extreme Team) to contribute chapters on the importance of eating and exercising your way into great skin.

As much as possible, this book will represent the same experience you would have if you come into my office to see me. We're working together as partners for your skin care health, and I have three passionate beliefs about skin care:

Knowledge heals. Throughout the book, I will explain what symptoms you can expect and what treatment will be like. It's simple—the more you know about what is happening (both on and under the surface of your skin), the better you'll be able to deal with it.

There's help and hope. I emphasize the widest range of solutions available, give you the specifics on my combination approach to skin healing, and outline treatment options that you can do at home or through your doctor's office. The goal is not just skin improvement but transformation.

The future will be better. In the pages that follow, you will find specific skin care regimens for your age, skin type, and condition. It's all aimed at one goal: to make your future better than your past.

In other words, your life never has to show on your skin again.

Behind the Scenes

YOUR ALL-ACCESS PASS
TO HOW SKIN WORKS

More than any other organ in your body, your skin is you. It gives an important first impression to people you meet through its appearance and expression. By being your physical contact with the world, it allows you to feel the velvety touch of a rose petal, the warm hug of a loved one, or a kiss. It also shows your heritage.

If you've purchased this book, are flipping through it in a bookstore, or are checking it out online, chances are you're facing some serious challenges with your skin. You might be dealing with flare-ups of adult acne, wrestling with the consequences of hormone changes from pregnancy to midlife, or struggling to offset the effects of illness as you work to reclaim your life.

Taking time to learn about how your skin functions may seem like a very low priority when your skin—not to mention your life—isn't working for you. But I'd like to ask you to stay with me and make the investment, for three critically important reasons:

Knowledge leads to success. The more you know about how your skin *should* function, the better we can collaborate on restoring it to its healthy, glowing best. I want to arm you with knowledge so that once you get through the immediate challenges you're facing, you'll be prepared for a future that's healthy, beautiful, and informed.

You're normal. It's no exaggeration to say that when you are dealing with serious skin challenges, you can start to feel like a pariah—isolated, abnormal, different from everyone else in a way that shows on your face. I want you to remember that you're none of these things. Your skin is simply responding the way it's designed to. There are lots of effective actions you can take to heal your skin within its very normal response range. Knowing how skin is programmed to defend itself—and recognizing just how infinitely broad the range of "normal" skin is, since every person's skin is unique—can be a huge confidence booster just when you need it most.

Skin is amazing. You can lose sight of this when your skin is under fire and is unrecognizable. I want you to know that your skin is a versatile, resilient, and marvelous "envelope." Getting to know your skin better will transform your skin from an enemy to an ally. I'd like to make you feel at home in your skin again and happy to be there.

In this chapter, you will:

- Get to know your skin and how it functions
- Understand the specifics of different ethnic skin types
- Learn about the powerful connection between healthy skin and the internal organs

An Amazing "Envelope"

If I were to ask you what your skin is, your first answer might be "a problem!" You may not recall that your skin is an organ: a bundle of functioning tissue, like your heart, your liver, and your brain. The skin is the largest, heaviest organ of the human body, and it performs many functions. On the average, we carry around twenty square feet of it, which weighs about six pounds. Over most of the surface of our bodies, the skin is only a few millimeters thick. It's thicker in places like the palms of our hands and the soles of our feet and is thinnest on our eyelids.

As surprising as it is to know what skin is, it's even more intriguing to look at what skin *does*.

The Function of the Skin

Most of the body's organs are specialists: each one does just one thing and does it well. Your skin, however, is an overachiever. It does many different things—some of them even contradictory—all at the same time.

Among the many items on your skin's to-do list every day are the following:

Contain everything. Your skin has what's known as an *integumentary* function. It's the "envelope" that surrounds and holds the body together mechanically. One of the most important things your skin contains is moisture: the water, blood, and other fluids that your body needs to stay alive.

Protect what's inside. Your skin is the body's first line of defense against the damaging effects of the elements. It serves as a barrier: a strong, waterproof seal against penetration by environmental poisons and harmful microorganisms.

Regulate your temperature. Your skin functions as an automatic thermostat, sensing changes in body temperature and interacting with your hypothalamus, the part of your brain that serves as an internal thermometer. When you're hot, your skin reacts by dilating (widening) your blood vessels, drawing warm blood away from the core of the body and toward the surface of the skin. Heat also triggers your skin to sweat. When the added moisture on the surface of your skin evaporates, it cools you down.

Fight disease and infection. Your skin contains a large range of cells that play a key role in immune response. These cells react to the presence of disease-producing viruses, fungi, and bacteria by triggering your body's internal defenses and sometimes killing them outright.

Make vitamin D. Most vitamins are not produced naturally by the body; they have to be ingested in food or as supplements. Vitamin D, which can be synthesized by the skin, is the exception.

Feel. The skin is a sensory organ. The exquisitely sensitive nerve endings in your skin react to heat, cold, pain, and pressure, serving as an early warning system or an amplifier of pleasure. Your skin can also show your feelings by responding to emotional sensations like anger, which causes flushing; embarrassment, which causes blushing; or happiness, which can create a rosy glow.

Express yourself. The skin reflects mood and internal health, but it also reflects our individual choices for self-presentation. In every human culture, cosmetics, tattooing, and even scarring of the skin, along with styling of the hair and nails, have been used as badges of identity and embellishments of personality. The specifics of what constitutes beauty may differ from age to age and place to place, but the attraction of beauty is universal—and skin is its ambassador.

Even when your skin is at its worst, as it may be right now, it continues to carry out as many of these vital functions as it can. Throughout this book I'll be helping you to support your skin while it's under siege so it can get back to doing what it does best.

The Structure of the Skin

THE SURFACE LAYERS

The skin that you can see and touch is just the tip of the skin's iceberg, the surface layer known as the *epidermis*. This outer protective layer is itself made up of several layers, each with its own specialized cells and activities.

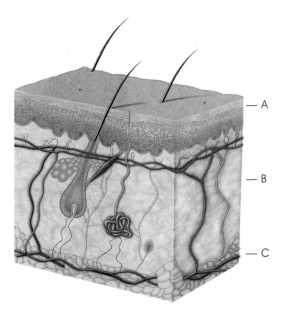

Cutaway diagram of the layers of skin:
(A) epidermis, (B) dermis, (C) subcutaneous tissue.

The Stratum Corneum

The outermost layer of the epidermis is called the *stratum corneum*. The stratum corneum is like the Great Wall of China—a barrier against outside threats. It is made up of flattened dead skin cells filled with a protein called *keratin*. (In a slightly harder form, keratin makes up our fingernails and toenails.) In addition, these cells form a tight seal to prevent loss of moisture through the skin. Oil glands between the cells of the stratum corneum manufacture lipids (moisturizing fats) to keep the skin supple and hydrated.

The keratinized cells of the stratum corneum are bound together by skin ceramides, natural lipids, and cholesterol. To illustrate, imagine that the cells are bricks in a wall and the ceramides, lipids, and cholesterol are the mortar holding them together. This mortar helps to create a physical barrier that is critical to maintain moist, well-hydrated skin.

When this mortar in the epidermis is affected by such factors as low humidity, harsh cleansers, declining estrogen levels, or chemotherapy, it changes so much that it can't function normally. The result is clumps of dry, dead skin cells on the surface of the skin. These dead cells build up unevenly and cling to the skin, giving it a dull, rough, scaly appearance. Compromised mortar also makes the skin more susceptible to irritation, opening up little fissures, allowing entry to viruses and bacteria. These little cracks in the wall are one more reason to maintain a moist and healthy stratum corneum, so that it can do its job as a barrier against intruders.

However, in healthy skin, these cells are shed one by one, invisibly. The dead cells of the stratum corneum are constantly being sloughed off in a process called *desquamation*, as living cells push upward from the lower layers of the epidermis. You lose thirty to forty thousand of these dead cells every minute of every day—nearly ten pounds a year—in a process that goes completely unnoticed, if all is working well.

It's this layer that we wash, moisturize, exfoliate, and make up—the part of our epidermis that is visible.

The Main Epidermis

Underneath the stratum corneum lies the body of the epidermis. There are four types of epidermal cells. The majority—about 95 percent—are called *keratinocytes*. They produce the protein keratin, which adds strength to the skin, the hair, and the nails. Also present in the epidermis are the following:

- **Melanocytes**   These are cells that manufacture melanin, the pigment that gives skin and hair their color.

The Life Cycle of Skin Cells

In the basement of the epidermis is a nursery, so to speak, where all of our epidermal skin cells are born and start life as stem cells. Stem cells are undifferentiated; they have the potential to become any kind of cell and carry out any kind of function. As they mature, these cells move upward through each layer of the epidermis, becoming more differentiated, or specialized, along the way.

By the time the cells reach the surface of the skin, they have fulfilled the majority of their functions. They flatten and die off, to be sloughed away. It takes about two weeks for a cell to travel from the "basement" to the middle of the epidermis, and then another four weeks to travel through the stratum corneum and be sloughed off. This cycle goes on continuously when your skin is healthy.

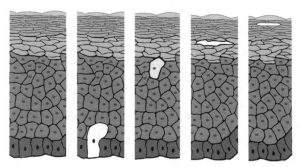

The life cycle of epidermal cells.

- **Langerhans cells**   These antigen–presenting cells are your body's first line of defense against microorganisms. They are also present in lymph nodes and alert other immune cells to combat infection.
- **Merkel cells**   These are sensory cells that respond to light touch and help your fingers to distinguish subtle differences in shape and texture.
- **Resident T cells**   Normal human skin contains about one million T cells per square centimeter. Recent studies have shown a role for these cells both in normal immunity and in inflammatory skin diseases such as psoriasis.

BENEATH THE SURFACE

There are two main layers beneath the epidermis: the dermis and the subcutaneous tissue.

DR. AVA'S SKINFORMATION

Skin-Color Differences

All skin structures are the same, no matter what the shade of your skin or your ethnicity. However, there are some significant differences:

- Asian skin has more sebaceous glands and more prominent melanocytes (the cells that manufacture melanin) compared to Caucasian skin.
- African American skin has a thicker stratum corneum but is more sensitive to irritants such as harsh soaps. It also has larger melanosomes (where the manufactured melanin is stored). These melanosomes give the skin its darker color and also contribute to post-inflammatory hyperpigmentation (PIH) at a site of inflammation, such as acne.
- Hispanic skin also has larger melanosomes, giving it greater propensity for PIH.
- African American skin has larger sebaceous glands.
- Caucasian skin has fewer and smaller sebaceous glands, smaller melanosomes, and a thinner stratum corneum than other groups.

The Dermis

Just below the epidermis is the skin's supportive layer, called the *dermis*. The thickness of the dermis, like that of the epidermis, varies in different parts of the body. Your dermal layer doubles in thickness twice in your life—once during your preschool years and again at puberty—and thins in later life. This infrastructure of the skin can be seriously affected by acne, hormonal changes, illness, and stress.

The dermis contains both cells and supporting proteins. *Fibroblasts* are the skin cells in the dermis that produce collagen, elastin, and other proteins and enzymes. The *extracellular matrix* surrounds the cells and serves as the scaffolding for the skin. It is chiefly composed of *collagen*, the fibrous protein that gives your skin its underlying structure. The extracellular matrix also contains *elastin*, the protein that gives your skin its ability to snap back after stretching, and *hyaluronic acid,* a complex sugar, which binds water, giving the dermis its volume. These three substances interact in a complex way to give your skin a moist, plump, and smooth youthful look. If you look at your face in a magnifying mirror, you'll notice more than skin. You'll see tiny hairs and the openings known as pores. You may notice a film of oil or drops of sweat on the surface of your skin. All of these come from the dermis's adnexal (conjoined) structures. A cross-section of the dermal layer shows the following:

- **Hair follicles** Every hair of the millions on your body emerges from a follicle, a tiny tube like the inverted finger of a glove.
- **Sebaceous glands** Connected to most hair follicles, these glands produce sebum, the oil that naturally moisturizes and helps to protect your skin.
- **Sweat glands** Also known as eccrine glands, these produce sweat that flows to the surface through their own ducts.

DR. AVA'S SKINFORMATION

The Difference between His Skin and Her Skin

Sex hormones are the main reason that men's skin and women's skin do not look and act the same. Lifestyle and grooming habits play a part, too. Here are some surprising facts:

- Men's skin is thicker than women's skin because it contains more of the structural proteins collagen and elastin.
- Women have more sweat glands than men, but men's sweat glands produce more sweat.
- Women have larger sebaceous glands than men, but men's sebaceous glands produce more oil.

- **Apocrine glands**   Present in some parts of the body, these scent glands are responsible for odor.

The dermis is also crowded with blood vessels that circulate nutrients to your skin, and nerves, which inform your skin about sensations like heat, cold, pain, itching, pressure, and touch.

The Subcutaneous Tissue

Underneath the dermis is the *subcutaneous* tissue, a layer of fat and connective tissue. Larger blood vessels and nerves run through this layer. Although technically not part of your skin, the subcutaneous tissue delivers nutrition and provides support to the dermis and the epidermis above.

Healthy Skin and Your Internal Organs

Just as there's a connection between good health and healthy skin, there's also an inside-outside dimension to the challenges your skin may face. As the largest organ of your body, your skin interacts in complex ways with every other physical system as well as your emotions. Your skin reflects what is going on inside your body, as in the expression "wearing your heart on your sleeve."

When your internal organs are functioning properly and are not undergoing stress from a disease or a stressful life condition, they function in congenial partnerships with the skin. When we experience a systemic illness such as rheumatoid arthritis, lupus, or diabetes, the initial symptom can be a rash on the skin. In fact, some of these rashes are diagnostic indicators of different forms of arthritis, of hormonal states, of vitamin deficiency (such as B_{12} anemia), or of hypothyroidism, to name a few.

Allergic reactions to internal medications can also manifest on the skin in the form of hives, dermatitis, swelling, and bumps. This intimate connection between the state of the internal organs and the skin exists because cells from the bloodstream course through the lymphatics (lymph vessels) in the skin.

One of the most significant relationships in the body exists between the hormones and the skin. The skin, like every other organ in the body, is deeply affected by hormonal surges, which can occur from neurological stimulation of the endocrine system: the adrenal glands, or the ovaries or testes. The central nervous system is stimulated by external pressures such as difficult life events and serious illness. It responds by attempting to ramp up the hormones that for millennia have been helpful in removing us quickly from stressful situations. The skin not only responds to external endocrine stimulation but is an endocrine organ in its own right. It performs this function in the hair follicle, where it converts testosterone to its active form, dihydrotestosterone (DHT). The DHT then acts directly on the sebaceous gland to secrete more sebum.

We can never overestimate the value of properly functioning skin to our overall health, nor can we ignore the connection between our internal state and the condition of our skin. When everything is working in harmony, your skin can feel like your best friend. When it's not, it's time to find out what's wrong and do everything you can to correct the problem.

In subsequent chapters, I'll go into the specifics of this inside-outside connection for adult acne, pregnancy, midlife skin, and the side effects of cancer treatments.

No matter how daunting skin challenges may seem, I want you to remember that almost all of these symptoms and effects are temporary—and every one of them is survivable. You can overcome a challenge by using the full range of skin, nutrition, and fitness solutions described here. You will regain, or even attain for the first time, the glowing vitality and sense of well-being that signal good health—and it will be written all over your face!

3

Enemies and Allies of the Skin

Everyone has enemies and allies. Sometimes we know their identities, and sometimes we can be fooled. Even your skin has them! The trick is learning how to enlist the allies and arm yourself against the enemies. The major enemies of the skin include free radicals, inflammation, glycation, and ultraviolet radiation. Other enemies of the skin are a poor diet, lack of exercise, lack of sleep, and the effects of chemotherapy. Although not an enemy, the major (and normal) hormonal swings experienced during pregnancy and menopause can also have an adverse impact on the skin.

All of these can wreak havoc on your skin and your internal organs in general. Some are the inevitable result of daily living, such as eating, breathing, and exposure to the environment. Fortunately, you do control some of these triggers, and their effect on the skin can be mitigated by lifestyle and diet changes. There are a number of allies available in your fight for better skin. These include diet, fitness, and good skin care.

Enemies of the Skin

Free Radicals

Free radicals, highly reactive molecules inside our bodies that can damage cell membranes, lipids, proteins, and DNA, are one major enemy of the skin. Even the simplest acts of breathing and eating create free radicals! They occur when oxygen is utilized to produce energy in our bodies. They are also created as our cells metabolize food for energy. They are "free" because each of them is an unpaired molecule searching for a partner.

The damage done by free radicals results in abnormal skin cells that are uneven, flat, and lacking in structural integrity rather than being even, round, and completely intact. The function of these skin cells is then compromised, which can eventually lead to wrinkles, lines, and brown spots because of decreased collagen production and altered pigment formation.

Although some free radicals are created through normal human metabolism, most of them are formed by external factors, such as ultraviolet exposure, smoking, air pollution, toxic chemicals, excessive alcohol consumption, and stress.

Free radicals are formed more readily as we age and when we are ill because our ability to neutralize them with our own naturally produced antioxidants declines. Fortunately, we can replenish our antioxidant stock by eating antioxidant-rich foods and applying topical antioxidant products.

Inflammation

When free radicals attack a cell, a cascade of enzymatic events occurs. Another enemy of the skin is unleashed: inflammation. Although inflammation is not usually visible to the naked eye (except for a sunburn, which makes the skin swollen and red), even low-grade inflammation is harmful, producing chemicals that accelerate the destruction of cells and disrupt their function.

Chronic inflammation can build up over time and result in numerous ailments, from problems that we can see, such as persistent acne, to more serious internal problems, such as heart disease. We can help to heal our skin by eating foods that are rich in anti-inflammatory ingredients and by applying anti-irritant, anti-inflammatory products to our skin.

Glycation

As delicious as sugar may seem to your taste buds, it can be extremely destructive to your skin. A spike in your blood sugar levels—which can come from eating processed foods or foods with too much refined sugar—can leave too much sugar circulating in your body. A process called *glycation* and the formation of *advanced glycation end products* are the results.

Glycation is a process whereby a sugar molecule, such as glucose or fructose, is added to collagen and elastin fibers, proteins found in the extracellular matrix, which surrounds skin cells. This makes the collagen stiff, as it is now cross linked in an abnormal way. In addition, the enzymes that normally remodel collagen no longer have access to the protein, and it can no longer be remodeled in a normal continual fashion. When this process occurs, the skin appears prematurely aged.

Glycation damages collagen in other organs in the body, too, including the blood vessel walls. When this occurs, the skin doesn't remodel in the same way as before, prematurely aging the tissue.

Ultraviolet Radiation

I purposely use the term *ultraviolet radiation* rather than *sun* when I name this enemy of healthy skin, because it's the ultraviolet (UV) part of the spectrum of sunlight that does the damage, and it's also present in tanning beds.

Yet although I use the term *radiation*, I'm not talking about the therapeutic uses of radiation, which may be part of your medical treatment plan. The most damaging radiation you may encounter in your life is found not in the nuclear medicine departments of hospitals but right outside your front door.

Ultraviolet radiation damage occurs from a combination of UVA and UVB waves, which penetrate both the Earth's ozone layer and your skin. The depth of penetration into the skin depends on the wavelength of the

UV ray in the light spectrum. UVA waves are considered long-wave at 320–400 nanometers (nm), and mid-wave UVB waves are about 280–320 nm. Both types of radiation deplete your skin's supply of protective antioxidants, which in turn leaves the skin open to further damage from sun exposure or disease.

Ultraviolet radiation damages the skin in two key ways:

- **UVB rays** cause visible changes in the skin. These rays absorb into the epidermis and are primarily responsible for freckling, tanning, and burning. We now know that these are not desirable souvenirs of a day at the beach or a session in a tanning bed. Rather, these skin changes are signs that the skin cells have sustained an injury, which can include DNA damage, immunosuppresion, and photoaging. Every exposure to UVB rays causes damage, even when it doesn't show up immediately.

   The naturally produced melanin in skin cells provides some protection from UVB rays, but without good sun protection the damage will still accumulate over time. Exposure to UVB radiation can decrease your skin's ability to fight off infection and adversely affect the immune function of the skin in other ways.

- **UVA rays** do not cause immediately noticeable damage. However, these are the rays responsible for photoaging in the long run. They penetrate more deeply into the skin than UVB rays and don't necessarily cause redness and burning. These rays damage the collagen itself and the collagen-producing cells at the dermal layer, gradually eroding the skin's infrastructure. With more exposure over time, this invisible insult becomes visible injury in the form of deep wrinkles and the potential for skin cancer.

Healthy Choices Are Your Allies

You may not have perfect control over your skin's enemies, but you can certainly enlist allies. The choices you make about your everyday behavior will directly affect—positively or negatively—your skin's present and future. Here are some of your allies in the quest to improve your skin health:

- **Eat an antioxidant-rich, anti-inflammatory diet.** Consuming whole foods—like lean poultry, fish, fruits, vegetables, nuts and seeds, and beans and whole grains—has been shown to improve acne by 50 percent, compared to processed and high-sugar foods, which promote inflammation and can disrupt blood sugar and insulin levels. Another major plus to a whole-foods, unrefined diet is that fresh produce is rich in antioxidants, which fight the inflammation that accompanies acne, hormonal changes, and cancer treatments including chemotherapy. (See chapter 5 for skin-healthy food choices.)

- **Control your stress.** Excess levels of cortisol—a hormone that is released when you're anxious, tense, or worried—affect your entire body, not only your skin. When the stress goes unchecked, the inflammation caused by cortisol simmers continuously, and the effects show on your face. Looking at your stressed-out face in the mirror brings on even more stress.

- **Adopt a skin care regimen and be consistent with it.** Faithfulness to a simple routine in the morning and the evening that cleanses, treats, and protects your skin is vital to healing your skin and maintaining its health.

- **Stay fit.** No matter what your level of general health may be or what physical challenges you face, there are ways to maintain an appropriate level of fitness. Exercising increases the oxygenation of your blood, which delivers nutrients to your skin. It also keeps you flexible and glowing and is a great stress-buster.

- **Get enough sleep.** Multiple studies have shown the importance of getting between seven and nine hours of uninterrupted sleep a night. It improves the function of your immune system, gives your body and skin time to repair themselves, and improves mental acuity.

- **Limit alcohol and avoid smoking or the use of drugs.** In addition to its other known serious health consequences, smoking damages your skin and speeds up the aging process. The toxic chemicals in cigarettes restrict circulation and create free radicals, which destroy collagen. Any toxin will increase inflammation, which in turn damages skin cells, collagen, and internal organs.

In short, the best way to be good to your skin is to be good to yourself.

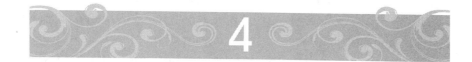

Building Your Skin Care Program

One of my patients, an actress who had just returned from filming a big movie in the South, told me how she learned the importance of following a good basic skin care program the hard way. "It was very hot, and we were on a tight shooting schedule with long hours," she said, "so I didn't always take the time to wash off my makeup every night. I started to break out."

Fortunately, she had packed one of my Radical Departure skin care products, which contains alpha-hydroxy acids to exfoliate dead cells as well as antioxidants to reduce inflammation and fight free radicals. After using the product regularly, she reported, "My skin became unbelievable. The texture returned to normal, the pores shrank down, and the bumps went away!"

I tell this story not to promote Radical Departure but to illustrate how adhering to a consistent skin care program with active ingredients will bring results: healthy, beautiful skin worthy of a movie star!

Switching skin care products constantly, leaving your makeup on at night, or skipping sunscreen will affect your skin's health and appearance. Cleansing, nourishing, and protecting your skin is even more vital if you also have adult acne or are facing any of the skin-related challenges associated with menopause or treatments for serious illnesses such as cancer. Your skin matters a lot—not just because right now it's calling for help, but also because it is so intimately connected to your inner and outer health, confidence, and beauty. Being good to your skin is a gift you give yourself that will outlast any health crisis.

It all starts with understanding the fundamentals of skin care. In this chapter, you will learn:

- The basics of good skin care
- Why it's important to practice good skin care
- How to choose and apply the right skin care products
- How to practice healthy skin care
- How to adjust your everyday skin care regimen so that your skin can always find its way back to being beautiful

The Basics of Good Skin Care

What is good skin care? It's actually very simple—using the right products and ingredients for your skin type, and using them consistently.

The first step involves determining your skin type. Again, I like to keep things simple. If you're not sure, choose the type that fits closest to your skin's "resting state" from the traditional three: oily, combination with T-zone, and dry. (Many skin-type charts also include a fourth type, so-called "normal" skin, but in my experience that's simply not a helpful category. Each person's skin is normal for them—and no one's skin is "normal," meaning completely issue-free all the time!)

Oily   If your skin often has a sheen and your pores jump out at you, most likely you have oily skin. You may have a tendency toward blackheads and whiteheads or breakouts, but you may also have fewer wrinkles than a lot of your friends of the same age.

Combination   If your skin feels oily in the T-zone—the T-shaped area that includes your forehead, nose, and chin—but your cheeks and jawline are normal or dry, you have combination skin.

Dry   Dry skin may feel tight or rough. You might see flaking, crinkling, or fine wrinkles. If you look in a magnifying mirror, you won't see many large pores; they're generally small and closed.

If you're still not sure of your skin type, take this quick test:

1. Wash your face with a gentle, nonfoaming cleanser and lukewarm water to remove any makeup, skin care products, or medications.
2. Rinse thoroughly and let your skin air-dry for fifteen to thirty minutes.
3. Blot your cheeks with a tissue. Use another tissue to blot the creases on each side of your nose.

If oil appears on both tissues, your skin is oily. If oil appears only on the tissue you used to blot your nose, you have combination skin with a T-zone. If no oil appears on either tissue and your face feels tight or itchy, you have dry skin.

In addition to your basic skin type, you will occasionally need to take other factors into account when designing your skin care program. These include the following:

Skin color   The degree of natural pigmentation in your skin affects how your skin responds to environmental insults, ranging from UV exposure to irritation and injury. Throughout this book I will explain how certain products and/or services might affect skin of color differently,

Sensitivity   The term *sensitive skin* has a wide range of meanings and implications, which is why I don't like to use it as a skin type category of its own. If you have dry skin, your skin may

> ## DR. AVA'S MYTH BREAKER
>
> **The myth:** Great skin is available in a jar—a really expensive jar.
>
> **The truth:** When it comes to healing your skin, there are miracles, but instant skin perfection, at whatever price, is not among them. Caring for your skin doesn't have to be complicated or expensive. This book includes all the information you'll need to get through many skin-related crises, but it all starts with the foundation of basic, good skin care habits outlined in this chapter.

be naturally more prone to irritation than it would be if your skin were oily. That is one type of sensitive skin. If your skin is oily, it can be more sensitive to pore-clogging ingredients that cause blemishes to form. If you have allergies or other conditions (whether systemic, like lupus, or skin-related, like eczema), you may be sensitive to particular substances or whole categories of ingredients. Finally, if you are undergoing treatment for a serious illness, your skin can become more sensitive to everything. Only you can judge your skin's sensitivity level, which is why I will always remind you to "listen" to your skin. Steer clear of products that make your skin uncomfortable.

The Building Blocks of Good Skin Care

Healthy skin makes you feel beautiful, and achieving it is not as complicated as you might think. To get good skin you need to cleanse, moisturize, nourish, and protect it every day. Think of these as the four basic building blocks of your skin care program.

Caring for your skin should become something you do automatically like brushing your teeth, once in the morning and once at night. And no, it won't take a lot of time. These few minutes at the beginning and end of each day are a mini spa treatment that will lift your spirits, improve your morale, and care for your skin. The best part is that if you make your skin care regimen a regular habit, you will see positive results quickly.

Morning

1. **Cleanse.** Starting the day with clean skin is the first step in keeping your skin fit and beautiful. If you start your day with a shower or bath, be sure to wash your face separately with the appropriate cleanser.
2. **Moisturize.** Your skin needs help to maintain its natural moisture content during the day. Moisturizing also gives you an opportunity to nourish your skin with antioxidants, peptides, and other nourishing ingredients.

3. **Protect.** We now know so much about how ultraviolet radiation from the sun harms skin—not only by triggering visible burns but also by affecting the skin's underlying structure. Both visible and invisible UV rays can damage the skin or lead to a serious illness, and not just on sunny days. As much as 60 percent of the sun's damaging radiation penetrates the clouds on even the grayest days. UVA rays, the kind that promote photoaging (wrinkles and brown spots), are not blocked by most windows. So put on sunscreen first thing in the morning and reapply it throughout the day.

   Sunscreen is especially vital when your skin is particularly vulnerable to UV damage. You may find that your skin is more vulnerable because of:

   Acne treatment   If you are using benzoyl peroxide, alpha-hydroxy acids (AHAs), beta-hydroxy acids (BHAs), or retinoids, your skin is being stripped of its natural protective layer of cells, and this makes it more vulnerable to UV radiation. Some oral antibiotics may also increase sensitivity to UV damage.

   Pregnancy or menopause   Estrogen swings can make your skin more vulnerable to UV damage.

   Cancer treatment   Chemotherapy and other targeted treatments increase the skin's susceptibility to UV damage. In the case of radiation therapy, the increased risk of skin disease and damage may be a permanent side effect in the treated area.

Evening

1. **Cleanse.** If you wear makeup, remove it before cleansing. If you wear waterproof mascara or eyeliner or very intense lip color, you may need products that are specifically designed to remove these before you wash your entire face.

   Note: Occasionally, your skin care routine may slip a little, especially when you are feeling very stressed. Try to never go to bed with your makeup on. That goes for mineral makeup, too, no matter what the manufacturer claims.

2. **Nourish/Treat.** Apply a serum with active ingredients such as retinoids, antioxidants, anti-inflammatories, or peptides that address your specific skin issues. They'll have time to do their work while

you sleep, when skin is in its reparative phase. (Retinoids also deteriorate quickly when exposed to light.). Serums should be applied before a moisturizer for best penetration.

Note: If you are using a topical prescription medication to treat acne or other skin condition, apply this to a freshly cleaned face before you apply anything else, unless your doctor has provided other instructions.

3. **Moisturize.** Your nighttime moisturizer can be a little richer and creamier than the daytime one you wear under sunscreen or makeup. Don't forget to moisturize your hands and feet at night, too, especially in the winter.

How to Choose and Apply Skin Care Products

Whether you're maintaining a daily skin care routine or need to develop one, it's good to understand how to choose the appropriate products to properly carry out your regimen. But you should never choose your skin care products based on an advertisement, the look of the jar, or its nice fragrance. You can find everything you need at reasonable prices in the personal products aisle of your local supermarket or drugstore. There are even many wonderful skin care products you can make in your own kitchen! (See chapter 11.)

Throughout this book I suggest ingredients to look for when you are purchasing skin care items. No matter what products you choose to use, the goal is healthy skin that is alive and luminous.

To give you a visual reference for quantities, I'm using pearls as the standard. The figure shows various sizes of pearls, pictured in their actual sizes.

Pearl sizes, shown in millimeters.

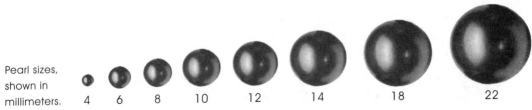

4   6   8   10   12   14   18   22

How to Choose a Cleanser

The purpose of a cleanser is to remove residue from your skin—external debris, natural secretions, and microorganisms. Choose a cleanser or a soap that is especially formulated for the face because they are gentler than those formulated for the body.

Cleansers come in a variety of forms:

- **Foaming cleansers** contain ingredients that generate lather. They are good at removing excess oil and dirt but can be drying or irritating to sensitive skin.
- **Nonfoaming cleansers** don't lather and are more soothing for sensitive, dry, or stressed skin. (Nondetergent cleansers, a subcategory of nonfoaming cleansers, are great for dry or sensitive skin but shouldn't be used if your skin is oily or acne-prone.)
- **Wipe-off cleansers** do not need to be rinsed, and come in forms such as cold creams, milky cleansers, or face wipes.

Cleansers often contain fragrance. When your skin is not under stress, you may enjoy using a naturally fragranced cleanser for its aromatherapeutic properties. If your skin is stressed, however, I recommend using fragrance-free cleansers, because the alcohol and oils associated with fragrance can be irritating to sensitive skin and may trigger allergic reactions even if you've never had a problem in the past.

Cleansers may also contain ingredients that address specific skin issues. Acne cleansers, for example, often include AHAs or BHAs to speed up the turnover of dead skin cells that can clog pores and cause blemishes. Cleansers formulated for mature or dry skin may contain moisturizers. Always choose one that best fits your skin profile.

Here are two signs that you may need to change your cleanser:

1. Your face is dry, irritated, red, or flaky.
2. After cleansing, your face feels greasy.

Overcleansing or using a product that is too drying can strip the skin of its protective sebum layer and lead to redness, inflammation, and dry, flaky skin. To determine what cleanser ingredients are best for your particular skin, check the skin care regimens at the end of chapters 6 through 9.

How to Wash Your Face

This section may seem obvious, but a good technique for skin cleansing is just as important as your choice of cleanser. To wash your face:

1. Pull your hair back so that it's easier to clean your whole face and neck. This way you won't transfer hair products to your clean skin.

2. Wet your face by splashing it gently with room-temperature water.

3. Put a dollop of cleanser about the size of a medium (14 mm) to large (18 mm) pearl (see the figure on page 30) into the palm of your wet hand. Rub your palms together to spread the cleanser evenly. Gently massage the cleanser onto your face, avoiding the eye area. Be sure to apply the cleanser about a quarter inch into your hairline to remove built-up hair products and to address any acne that may be present in these areas. Don't forget to cleanse under your chin and the back of your neck.

4. Rinse thoroughly by splashing your face or by using a clean, wet washcloth.

5. Pat—don't rub—your skin dry with a clean cotton towel. If your skin is particularly dry or sensitive, leave your skin damp. Applying moisturizer to skin that's slightly wet improves absorption of active ingredients and seals in the moisture.

In the evening, remove your makeup before cleansing. Use a premoistened pad or a disposable wipe formulated for gentle makeup removal and tailored to your skin type. Don't leave behind any waterproof mascara that might irritate your eyes. And remember, when you are in the shower, wash your face last—after you have rinsed off any shampoo or conditioner.

How to Choose a Moisturizer

This is the most frequently asked question in my practice. We demand a lot from our moisturizers. They are expected to relieve dry sky, repair signs of aging (such as fine lines, wrinkles, and brown spots), and work with prescription medications that are used to treat a multitude of skin conditions. Fortunately, there is now an enormous range of moisturizers that can meet our expectations. The tricky part is selecting one that is appropriate for your particular needs.

Your choice of moisturizer should be tailored to your skin type as follows:

- **Water-based** is better for oily or acne-prone skin.
- **Oil-based** is better for dry, mature, or sensitive skin.

Moisturizers also come in various formulations that are appropriate for different skin types. The most common are:

- **Gel:** slippery; appropriate for oily or combination skin
- **Lotion:** fluid and light; appropriate for all skin types
- **Cream:** thick and rich; appropriate for dry skin
- **Ointment:** very thick; only for extremely dry skin

You want your moisturizer to absorb into the skin and make your skin feel slightly moist and supple. Moisturizers that slide off your face on a hot day or land on your pillow overnight won't do you much good. To test whether a particular formulation will absorb well into your skin, lightly massage a few drops on the back of your hand and wait a minute or two. If it feels sticky or greasy or remains very slick, the formulation is too thick for your skin. If it has vanished completely, and your skin feels dry or tight, it's too thin or light.

There are three basic moisturizing components, and each performs a slightly different job when it comes to skin care.

ASK DR. AVA

My skin is very sensitive. Is it better for me to choose products that contain all-natural ingredients?

Natural ingredients are less likely to trigger allergic reactions than their synthetic counterparts. If you have existing allergies or sensitivities to certain substances, however, make sure that they're not included—in natural or synthetic form—in the products you use. Plant families can also trigger allergic reactions. For example, if you have seasonal allergies triggered by goldenrod pollen, it's best to stay away from products containing chamomile, a related plant.

1. **Humectants** attract water from the dermis into the epidermis and prevent skin from losing moisture from the "outside in." Humectants include glycerin, lactic acid, urea, hyaluronic acid, sorbitol, and honey.

2. **Occlusives** block evaporation of moisture through the skin's surface. They also act as emollients, or skin softeners, and include mineral oils, petroleum jelly, zinc oxide, lanolin oil, and silicons.

3. **Emollients** add lubrication to the surface of the skin by filling the spaces between skin flakes to make the texture smoother and softer. These include jojoba oil, shea butter, olive oil, squalene, fatty acids, and rosehip oil.

If your skin is under stress, pick a moisturizer with ingredients that address your particular skin issue:

- Acne medications tend to be very drying, so counterbalance them with a light moisturizer that contains antioxidants to reduce inflammation.
- To help with the roller-coaster effect of hormonal changes during pregnancy, pick a moisturizer with soothing properties and anti-inflammatories. While pregnant, you may need to use a moisturizer on areas of your body where you didn't need one before.
- Help your menopausal skin compensate for the effects of estrogen depletion by adding extra moisturizers with active ingredients that stimulate collagen repair. A gentle, all-over moisturizer will be one of your best defenses.

At the end of chapters 6 through 9 are detailed lists of ingredients for each skin type and skin condition covered in that chapter.

Key Ingredient Categories

It is beneficial to follow a skin care regimen that includes active ingredients that are appropriate for your skin type. Important groups include anti-inflammatories, antioxidants, retinoids, and peptides.

Anti-inflammatories   Anti-inflammatories are often plant-derived and can help the skin heal on the surface and at the cellular level, where the inflammatory process takes place. These extracts, known as polyphenols, often do double duty as antioxidants and include soy isoflavones and extracts of grape seed, green tea, licorice, and rosemary.

Antioxidants   No matter what your skin type, antioxidants are some of the most important ingredients you can have in your skin care arsenal. These scavenge for harmful free radicals, brighten the skin, and unify its color. Some of the most popular antioxidants are vitamins A, C, and E, along with alpha-lipoic acid, coffeeberry, resveratrol, coenzyme Q10, and idebenone. Current research shows that combinations of different antioxidants have a synergistic effect, which gives a better outcome than the use of one antioxidant alone.

Alpha hydroxy acid   Derived from fruit, milk, and sugars, alpha hydroxy acid (AHA) is an exfoliant that assists with cell turnover to even out skin tone. AHA is reported to improve wrinkling, roughness, pigmentation, and photodamage. Commonly used AHAs include glycolic acid, lactic acid, citric acid, malic acid, and tartaric acid.

Beta hydroxy acid   Beta hydroxy acid (BHA) works as a "degreaser" and an exfoliant, causing dead cells of the epidermis to slough off, allowing for regrowth of new skin. BHA can dissolve oil and dead-skin buildup in pores, which can prevent the formation of blackheads and blemishes. The most common BHA is salicylic acid.

Botanicals   Extracts from fruits, vegetables, and plants have a variety of anti-inflammatory and anti-irritant properties. They are used to accelerate epidermal barrier function repair, reduce discoloration, reverse photodamage, and assist in skin healing, among other functions. Botanicals include ginkgo biloba, green tea, aloe vera, chamomile, calendula, soy, papaya, witch hazel, and mushrooms.

Ceramides   Ceramides replenish the lipids of the skin's stratum corneum and are critical to the barrier properties of the skin.

Epidermal growth factor   Epidermal growth factor (EFG) is a complex family of hormones

DR. AVA'S SKIN SAVERS

Always test moisturizers and other skin care products before you buy them. You can request samples from manufacturers online or from skin care consultants in salons, department stores, and beauty supply centers. Drugstores and discount retailers may display sample containers or allow you to test products if you ask. Your dermatologist's office is another place to turn for skin care product samples and consultation.

produced by the body to control cell growth and division. Adding some forms of EGF to your skin care regimen may assist with skin remodeling, reverse photoaging, and treat wrinkles.

Peptides These are chains of amino acids that are the building blocks of skin's collagen. With consistent use, some peptides have shown to significantly reduce fine lines and wrinkles and produce younger-looking skin. They also can prevent the irritation that is common with the use of retinoids. Peptides include palmitoyl pentapeptide, acetyl hexapeptide, and neuropeptide.

Probiotics These are the "friendly" bacteria that fight the "bad" bacteria that cause acne and eczema.

Retinoids These are derived from vitamin A and vary from prescription-strength retinoic acid to over-the-counter retinols. They have anti-oxidant properties and promote collagen production, reduce brown spots and wrinkles, firm the skin, and can treat acne. They are a great addition to an evening skin care regimen.

Stem cells Apple stem-cell extract is a new ingredient derived from the stem cells of a rare Swiss apple. Several studies have shown that these stem cells stimulate human-skin stem cells to proliferate, thereby increasing the life span of fibroblasts, which make the collagen that adds fullness to our skin. This extract may be of value to skin that's been subjected to harsh stressors like chemotherapy.

Vitamins These help restore photodamaged skin and have other anti-aging properties. Certain vitamins also help hydrate the skin. Vitamin E protects from ultraviolet light damage and increases the efficacy of sunscreen ingredients. Vitamin C reduces inflammation and prevents water loss. Vitamin B_5 improves skin elasticity and reduces roughness. Vitamin K addresses undereye circles and mitigates skin bruising.

How to Apply a Moisturizer

Apply moisturizer after cleansing, exfoliating, and applying optional eye cream, serum, or prescription medication—but before putting on your sunscreen or makeup. If your skin is very dry or sensitive, apply moisturizer while your skin is still damp from cleansing or showering.

To apply moisturizer:

1. Put a dollop of moisturizer the size of a medium pearl (10 mm to 14 mm) in the palm of your hand. Rub your palms together to spread the moisturizer evenly, and gently massage onto your face. If you have oily skin or combination skin with a T-zone, you can apply moisturizer just to the drier parts. If your skin is dry, apply moisturizer evenly over your entire face, with the exception of the area around your eyes.
2. You may apply moisturizer to your neck and upper chest. The skin in these areas contains fewer oil glands, sweat glands, and hair follicles than the skin on your face, and can be especially sensitive and subject to dryness.
3. Wait a minute or two for your skin to absorb the moisturizer before applying sunscreen and makeup.

How to Choose a Serum

Serums are fluid products with high concentrations of ingredients such as vitamins, antioxidants, and peptides designed to nourish and repair your skin. Serums can be water- or oil-based. Because they are made of small molecules, they can deliver ingredients deeper into the skin. They are usually applied before any other skin care products, such as moisturizers. Serums address a variety of skin concerns including rejuvenation, dehydration, inflammation, and discoloration.

How to Apply a Serum

Apply serum after cleansing your face but before applying moisturizer or prescription topical medications, unless otherwise directed by your dermatologist.

1. After patting your skin dry, put a small pearl-size amount (6 mm to 8 mm) of product on your fingertips.
2. Use your fingertips to apply the serum all over your face, gently massaging it into your skin. Don't forget your neck and chest.

3. Immediately, you can follow with a moisturizer or other topical skin care product such as another serum. Yes, serums can be layered on the face.

Some serums can be applied around the eye area, but make sure to read the label before doing so.

Protecting Your Skin from the Sun

Protecting your skin from the sun is the most important step you can take to prevent premature aging, wrinkles, discoloration, and skin cancer. It is especially crucial when your skin is vulnerable from adult acne, hormonal changes, or chemotherapy. There are many products to choose from, so here is your Sun Protection 101:

UVA, UVB, and UVC   The sun emits ultraviolet radiation that is classified into UVA, UVB, and UVC rays. Most UVC is absorbed by the ozone layer and does not reach Earth.

UVB rays are the main cause of skin reddening and sunburn. They tend to damage the skin's more superficial, epidermal layer. UVB intensity varies by season, location, and time of day. However, UVB rays can damage your skin all year, especially at high altitudes or if there is a reflective surface involved, such as snow or ice. UVB rays play a major role in the development of skin cancer and photoaging.

UVA rays account for up to 95 percent of the UV radiation that reaches Earth's surface. They are thirty to forty times more prevalent than UVB rays, are present during all daylight hours all year, and can penetrate clouds and glass. This means that even while sitting in your car or office, you are exposed to UVA rays.

UVA protection   There is currently no accepted rating system in the United States for determining whether a product provides UVA protection. However, many products have been tested for UVA protection, and it is important to look for a brand that contains Helioplex, Mexoryl, zinc oxide, or titanium dioxide.

Sun Protection Factor   Sun Protection Factor (SPF) is *not* an amount of protection, per se, but rather a laboratory measure of the effectiveness of sunscreen. The higher the SPF, the more protection the sunscreen offers against UVB. The SPF is the amount of UV radiation needed to cause sunburn on skin with the sunscreen on. So if you are wearing sunscreen with SPF 30, for example, your skin will not burn until it has been exposed to 30 times the amount of solar energy that would normally cause it to burn. The problem with these ratings is that they are inexact. Most people fail to apply the same amount of sunscreen that was used when the product was tested in a lab. In fact, we generally apply only one quarter of the amount that is used during product testing. We tend to apply sunscreen unevenly, leaving some areas of the skin unprotected. You cannot strictly rely on a product's SPF to guarantee that you are totally protected from the sun.

Regardless of the SPF, I always recommend that you apply *two* coats of sunscreen—include your nose, lips, hands, neck, ears, and chest—and reapply frequently if you are swimming, sweating, washing, or doing anything that could cause your sunscreen to rinse off.

Sunscreen   Sunscreen contains active chemicals such as avobenzone and padimate that absorb, reflect, or scatter ultraviolet rays and prevent them from penetrating the skin. Sunscreen absorbs UVB rays and may filter out some UVA rays.

Sunblock   Sunblock contains ingredients that physically block the sun's rays from reaching the skin by reflecting as well as dispersing them, much the same way a mirror would. Sunblock uses one of only two active ingredients: titanium dioxide or zinc oxide. The ingredient with the widest protective absorption spectrum in the UVA and UVB

ASK DR. AVA

I am very fair-skinned. Is it worth it for me to use a sunscreen with a very high SPF like 85, or is there no real extra protection at that point?

There has been an increased tendency to recommend higher SPF products (over 30), especially for people with fair or sensitive skin. A recent study has shown that because we underapply sunscreen, higher SPF sunscreens give a margin of safety and may provide more effective protection. Fewer "sunburn" cells, markers of UV-induced DNA damage, are seen in fair-skinned people who use higher SPFs.

range available in the United States is zinc oxide. In the past, sun-blocks were sticky, white, and pasty. They have now been micronized for easy, elegant application.

Broad spectrum   A product with this label combines ingredients that provide protection from both UVA and UVB rays. Broad-spectrum sunscreens generally require at least three active ingredients, which may include PABA derivatives, salicylates, and/or cinnamates (octyl methoxycinnamate and cinoxate) to absorb UVB rays; benzophenones (such as oxybenzone and sulisobenzone) for shorter-wavelength UVA protection; and avobenzone (Parsol 1789), ecamsule (Mexoryl), titanium dioxide, or zinc oxide for the remaining UVA spectrum.

How to Choose Sun Protection

Now that you know your sun protection basics, here are my tips for choosing the best product for you:

Choose a broad-spectrum sunscreen with an SPF of at least 30. Alternately, choose a sunblock based on what works best for your skin and your amount of UV exposure. If your sun protection product is uncomfortable or messy, you won't use it. Test the absorbency of sun protection products on the back of your hand. Think about whether you'll need a waterproof product, which can be sticky, or one that goes on dry so that makeup application is easier.

Know your ingredients. A number of sunscreens now have antioxidants as additives. Because some ultraviolet rays penetrate even the best sunscreen, these antioxidants can support the skin to prevent UV damage. Some common antioxidants are vitamin C, green tea extract, pomegranate, and beta-carotene.

ASK DR. AVA

I've heard that if I get enough of certain antioxidants from nutrition and supplements, I won't need to use sunscreen. Is it true that there are more natural ways to protect the skin from the effects of UV radiation?

Some studies have shown that antioxidant nutrients like beta-carotene, lutein, lycopene, and omega-3 fatty acids can enhance the skin's ability to withstand the damaging effects of sun exposure. However, I stress *enhance* because oral or topical antioxidants don't replace good, careful sun protection. Getting lots of antioxidants in your diet—preferably through fresh whole foods—will promote good health throughout your body, including your skin, and will add to the good sun protection habits you should also be practicing.

Experiment with various formulations. Sunscreens are available as powders, lotions, gels, and sprays, and in a waxy base like a Chapstick. Choose one that is comfortable to wear, that is not too sticky, and that gives you good coverage. If your sunscreen triggers a breakout, switch brands. Sometimes the rash is not from the sunscreen but from what is called *prickly heat*, which occurs when your sweat glands can't properly drain. If this occurs, see your health care provider to find out what is causing your rash.

> **DR. AVA'S SKINFORMATION**
>
> Some studies have shown that uncoated yellow oxide and black oxide pigments in mineral makeup can degrade the avobenzone in a sunscreen formula, making it ineffective. If you wear mineral makeup, check to make sure that the pigments are coated, or choose a sun protection product without avobenzone.

Remember that no sunscreen is truly waterproof. Before 2002, sunscreens were often labeled water-resistant—defined by the Food and Drug Administration (FDA) as requiring reapplication after forty minutes of exposure to water or sweat—or waterproof, defined by the FDA as lasting for eighty minutes before requiring reapplication. Since 2002, however, the FDA has prohibited the use of the term *waterproof* as misleading, because all sun protection products must be reapplied at some point after you've been in the water.

How to Apply Sun Protection

Sun protection is one of the most misapplied products in basic skin care. In the following steps, I've highlighted the things you need to remember so you can correct your practice if necessary or build correct habits from the start:

1. Apply sunscreen or sunblock after moisturizing, unless your moisturizer contains a sunscreen. Apply it at least thirty minutes before going outside.
2. In order to be sure that you get enough coverage, use a higher SPF.
3. Apply sunscreen or sunblock evenly to all exposed skin—not just your face, but into your hairline (and on your scalp if your hair doesn't cover it), on the tips of your ears, on your neck (including the nape), on your chest, and on the backs of your hands. Individ-

uals with dark skin must also use sunscreen or sunblock, because they are still at risk for sun damage and melanoma.

4. Reapply sunscreen every two hours when you're in the sun and more frequently if you sweat or swim. If you remove and reapply makeup during the day, reapply sunscreen before reapplying makeup.

5. Use full-spectrum sun protection lip balm if you'll be outdoors.

6. Increase your level of sun protection when your skin is particularly sensitive to UV radiation: when you are pregnant, when you're taking medications (such as hormone replacement therapy) that cause photosensitivity, or when you are dealing with a serious illness.

Other Sun Protection Strategies

Because no form of sunscreen can provide 100 percent protection from all UV exposure, do your skin a favor by employing extra protective measures, especially when your skin is under siege:

- Wear a hat made of tightly woven material that has a brim at least five inches deep all the way around.
- Cover up with SPF-rated clothing that filters UV rays.
- Wear sunglasses or snow goggles with full-spectrum UV protective lenses; large wraparound styles offer the best protection.
- Stay out of direct sunlight (even coming through windows or on shaded patios) as much as possible.
- Remember that water and snow reflect and intensify UV radiation.
- Check your blood levels of vitamin D with your physician to see if you need to take a supplement.

Skin Care Multitasking

You can simplify your basic skin care program by choosing products that do double duty. Here are some common combinations:

- Combine cleansing and exfoliating by using a cleanser that contains AHAs or gentle scrubbing ingredients.

- Offset the drying or irritating effects of some acne medications by blending them with a little moisturizer before applying, or apply the medication after lightly moisturizing your skin.
- On days that you won't be outside or directly exposed to UV radiation, choose a daytime moisturizer that contains a full-spectrum sunscreen.
- You can skip foundation or concealer by using a tinted moisturizer that is compatible with your skin tone.

Expanding Your Skin Care Program

Depending on your skin's particular needs and your own preferences, you may want to expand your "cleanse, moisturize, nourish, and protect" skin care program to include additional steps. This can include the use of exfoliants, toners, eye creams, masks, scrubs, and peels.

To get the most effective use of your products, use them in this order:

Daily Expanded Skin Regimen
- Cleanser
- Exfoliant
- Toner
- Eye cream
- Serum/Nourish/Treat
- Moisturizer
- Sun protection

Biweekly Expanded Skin Regimen
- Scrub or Mask: use after cleansing, and follow with your regular regimen

Exfoliant

Gentle exfoliation can be part of your daily cleansing routine. It helps maintain the healthy growth and turnover cycle of the skin's outer layer, the epidermis. Exfoliation removes dead skin cells and promotes better circulation. It can be beneficial to many areas of your body, including your face, arms, legs, and feet. There are different approaches for each area, and certain exfoliation techniques work best with certain skin types.

There are two basic types of exfoliants: physical and chemical. Physical exfoliants work to remove dead skin cells via friction. This can include simply rubbing your face with a moistened washcloth. With chemical exfoliants it is the chemical, not the friction, that does the job. Most chemical exfoliants found in facial cleansers are mild acids, such as salicylic acid. They exfoliate by dissolving the "glue" that binds dead skin cells to other skin cells.

Over-the-counter exfoliants should contain neither fragrance nor color, which may irritate sensitive skin. Never exfoliate if your skin is irritated from inflamed acne, rosacea flares, or a skin-related illness. Skin of color may overreact to exfoliation by changing pigment, so check with your dermatologist before including it in your skin care regimen. However, if your skin is under stress from acne flares or has been made vulnerable by chemotherapy, even the gentlest exfoliation may be too much. And never exfoliate around the eye area—-the skin is very sensitive and can be easily damaged.

To exfoliate:

1. Wash your face, as described in the previous section.
2. Take a medium to large amount of exfoliant—about the size of a medium (14 mm) to large (22 mm) pearl—and gently apply it to your damp skin. The key word is *gently*.
3. Massage the exfoliant over your skin. Never press it into your skin. Remember, you are not sanding wood, and you don't get extra points for strength! Avoid the delicate eye area. You can also exfoliate your neck and chest, but you must be very gentle.
4. Use a washcloth dampened with warm water to wipe off the exfoliant.
5. Apply your skin care products.

Toner

Many people find that toners make their skin feel clean and fresh compared to just using a cleanser. Toners can also help rebalance the pH of your skin and penetrate pores more deeply than some cleansers. Toners can be referred to as astringents, tonics, clarifiers, and facial mists. It's a popular misconception that toners can shrink your pores or tone your skin. However, they do help remove extra residue and are an extra step in washing your face. Toners should never make your face feel tight or sore.

If you like the feel of a toner, make sure that it adds value to your basic skin care plan. Toners can:

- Deliver antioxidants
- Hydrate the skin
- Control oil production
- Soothe after cleansing
- Help reduce inflammation

Astringents are alcohol-based toners that may contain salycilic acid and are often used for oily, acne-prone skin. Use them with caution, as they can be irritating and drying to your skin, especially when your skin is under stress.

Witch hazel and distilled rosewater are gentle, natural toners that have anti-inflammatory properties and a refreshing quality.

To apply a toner:

1. Cleanse and gently pat dry your face.
2. Moisten a cotton pad with a generous amount of the toner.
3. Apply the cotton pad in a sweeping motion across your face.
4. To use a spray toner, lightly mist your face from a short distance until your face is damp.
5. Immediately follow use of the toner with serum and/or moisturizer and sun protection.

DR. AVA'S SKINFORMATION

You can make your own rosewater by steeping rose petals (preferably with a deep color and scent, from organically grown rosebushes) in very hot distilled water for about forty-five minutes. Let the mixture cool, then strain it through cheese-cloth into a sterilized glass container with a lid. Homemade rosewater will keep a day or two at room temperature or longer in the refrigerator.

Eye Cream

The eye area has the thinnest and most sensitive skin on the body, and various products have been designed to combat fine wrinkles, puffiness, dark circles, and crepey or dehydrated skin.

Eye creams are designed specially to treat the delicate skin in this area and migrate into the eye itself. There are two main types of eye creams.

1. **Day cream** is designed to enhance the appearance of your eyes during the day and may contain SPF.
2. **Night cream** is designed to help repair and prevent further damage to your skin. (AHA and/or retinol are common ingredients.)

When choosing an eye cream, always pick one with ingredients targeted to your particular issue. For example, if you want an eye cream to combat dark circles, look for one that contains vitamin K, kojic acid, and hydroquinone. If you prefer an eye cream with more firming properties, look for one that contains caffeine, retinol, AHA, copper, and vitamin C.

To apply eye cream:

1. Place a very small amount—about the size of a seed pearl (4 mm to 6 mm)—of eye cream on the tip of your finger.
2. Below your eye, dot the cream along the eye socket bone from the outside corner in toward your nose. Above your eye, dot the cream only along the brow bone, avoiding the eyelid itself to prevent the cream from getting into your eye.
3. Pat the area around the eye repeatedly to ensure that the cream you initially spread is absorbed into the skin. This is done very gently.
4. Wait a few minutes before putting on your eye makeup to give the cream time to set. Many eye creams provide a good base for eye makeup or undereye concealer, keeping them from caking or smearing.

Masks, Scrubs, and Peels

Your skin care program may include the occasional use of a mask, scrub, or peel. These can be used to address specific skin issues or just to give you the luxury of an at-home facial treatment. They can be purchased already prepared, or you can make your own, using the recipes I've provided in chapter 11. Make sure the ingredients are appropriate to your skin type and/or condition, especially if you have acne flares, rosacea, or eczema. You may need to talk to your dermatologist before using these kinds of products.

- Masks generally use mineral or botanical ingredients in a solution that's applied to the skin and allowed to dry, then rinsed off. You can also purchase paper or microfiber masks that have been imbued with the ingredients; you simply moisten the mask and place it on your face.
- Scrubs may be used as occasional extra exfoliation. Most scrubs consist of mildly abrasive particles—botanical, mineral, or synthetic—suspended in a cleansing or a moisturizing base. Scrubs are massaged into the skin and then thoroughly rinsed off.
- Peels involve a product that is applied to the face and allowed to dry into a film that can be peeled away. These can range from intensive peels performed by a professional to at-home peels you can apply yourself.

When to See a Dermatologist

If you find that your existing skin care regimen is not working, if you still have skin issues even after adjusting your regimen, or if you simply are not sure how to take care of your skin, you may need to seek the help of an experienced dermatologist. A dermatologist can provide specialized medical care and offer reparative and cosmetic skin treatments. Ask your physician or other health care provider for referrals. Don't hesitate to seek out a doctor who understands your particular skin care issues.

Understanding Product Labels and Claims

Reading labels on skin care products can be confusing. How much of a particular ingredient does a product contain? Are there any ingredients *not* listed on the label that might be potentially harmful? The FDA requires that skin care product ingredients be listed, but it doesn't require the manufacturer to reveal the amounts or concentrations by percentage. To see how ingredients are listed, look at the sample labels in the appendix. Here's how to know what you're getting:

- Ingredients are listed in order from the highest concentration to the lowest.
- Use the rule of thirds. The top third of the ingredients list makes up about 90 percent of the product. The middle third is responsible for 8 to 9 percent. The bottom third of the ingredients makes up only 1 to 2 percent of the product. One exception is that any ingredient classified as a drug by the FDA, such as Retin-A or benzoyl peroxide, will be listed either first (no matter what its concentration) or in a separate "active ingredients" list. Most manufacturers will provide concentration percentages for active ingredients.
- Ingredients you pay a premium for, such as peptides, ceramides, or vitamin C, should be listed in the top third, or you're not getting enough to matter, even if the product label and advertising feature the ingredient prominently.
- Ingredients listed in the bottom third are usually present in trace amounts. This means that beneficial ingredients aren't present in concentrations large enough to have any effect. Conversely, trace ingredients that may be irritating or even toxic at higher concentrations are not present in concentrations high enough to be harmful.
- Know that manufacturers may use the popular or the scientific (usually Latin or Greek) names for ingredients. Water may be listed as aqua, and vitamin E may appear as tocopherol. To know what you're getting, look up the ingredient names online.
- Watch for ingredients that may trigger any kind of sensitivity or allergic reaction. If you have a gluten allergy, for example, avoid wheat germ. People with hay fever or seasonal allergies often react to chamomile. Low concentrations applied topically may not be problematic unless your skin is under stress.
- Many ingredients listed on a label can be included for purposes other than actively caring for your skin. They help to make the product smoother, add fragrance or color, prolong shelf life, or protect the product from bacterial or fungal contamination.

Now that you understand how skin care prod-ucts list their ingredients, what about their claims? Are they always true? Are they ever true? Because skin care products (with the exception of prescrip-tion medications) are not regulated by the FDA, any claims made on their labels have not been verified by an independent agency. Use common sense. The more miraculous the claim, the more skeptical you should be. You're reading marketing copy, not med-ical charts. Here are some common terms and what they do (and don't) mean:

Alcohol-free means that the product is free of ethyl alcohol. However, it still may contain fatty alcohols, such as cetyl or stearyl alcohol, which serve as moisturizers.

Non-comedogenic means that the manufacturer claims the product will not clog pores or cause acne flares. There are no FDA standards for this claim, however. To be safe, interpret it as meaning "may be less likely to trigger breakouts than some other products."

Hypoallergenic means the manufacturer claims the product will be less likely to cause allergic reactions in sensitive people. There are no FDA standards for this claim either. You should always use your own discretion about which products may be likely to trigger a reaction. For example, if you don't usually have sensitive skin, but you are dealing with cancer treatments, stress, or acne, hypoallergenic products might provide an extra level of gentleness.

Natural is an advertising term and has no FDA definition. Many chemical ingredients are as natural as botanicals and less irritating. If you like the idea of buying natural products, look for botanical ingredients in high concentrations.

Organic has a legal definition in the United States. Growers of organic agricultural products (like the botanicals used in some skin care products)

ASK DR. AVA

My skin is dry, and I'm trying to avoid products containing alco-hol. When I check the ingredients list on products labeled alcohol-free, however, I see several different kinds of alcohol listed. How can that product be labeled alcohol-free?

Not all alcohols are the same. The kind we want to avoid in skin care products is ethyl alcohol and its relatives, like isopropyl (rubbing) alcohol. These are too drying for dry or sensitive skin. However, there are good alco-hols—the so-called fatty alcohols, such as cetyl alcohol or stearyl alcohol—that actually help your skin retain moisture. They are derived from coconut and other similar plant oils or are chemically synthesized. Products labeled alcohol-free are free of drying alcohols but may include other alcohols.

must meet strict standards, including refraining from the use of chemical fertilizers and pesticides. In order for a product to be labeled organic, it must contain no less than 95 percent certified organic ingredients. Products made with 70 percent organic ingredients may be advertised as "made with organic ingredients."

The products in both of these categories will carry the U.S. Department of Agriculture (USDA) Organic seal. If a product is made with less than 70 percent organic materials, it may not be labeled or advertised as organic, but the individual organic ingredients may carry an asterisk with the note "certified organic" in the ingredients list.

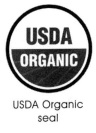

USDA Organic
seal

Not tested on animals or *cruelty-free* may be used by manufacturers to claim that the particular product or formulation has not been tested on animals or that the company itself conducts no animal tests. However, individual ingredients that go into a product may have been animal-tested at some point. There are no FDA standards governing the use of these terms.

Conclusion

No matter what else is going on in our lives, we always want our skin to look beautiful. The easiest way to get and keep great skin is to adopt a basic skin care program now. No, it doesn't have to be complicated. As I said before, it just has to be consistent and include excellent sun protection. You can use any products from any product line you choose, whatever best fits your skin type and your particular needs.

Stay flexible. The products and techniques you use to care for your skin will change as you change, especially if you're facing one or more of the skin challenges this book addresses.

Good Nutrition

HEALING YOUR SKIN FROM THE INSIDE OUT

Advice from Wendy Bazilian, Dr.P.H., R.D.
and Ava Shamban, M.D.

n this chapter, you will learn about:

- The connection between good nutrition and healthy skin
- The importance of nutrients and superskin foods
- Shifting your eating habits to an anti-inflammatory diet
- Meal plans to help you eat your way to a lifetime of great skin

Few people realize that eating well is easy and satisfying and that it will almost immediately improve your skin's complexion, tone, moisture, elasticity, and overall vibrancy.

You can practically eat your way to better skin. But it's not only your skin that thrives on good nourishment from real food; your whole body does, too. Plus, you get to enjoy eating great, delicious food. We call that a win-win-win.

The Foundation: A Balanced Diet

A healthy diet and healthy skin are closely linked. A balanced diet promotes good health and longevity. It helps to prevent disease and counteracts the abuses of exposure to pollution, UV rays, chemicals, stress, and the effects of regular daily living.

Your skin needs good nourishment, too—constant, regular input from a healthy diet to help it regenerate and thrive. A nutritious diet provides the nutrients that are necessary for your skin's cells. When your skin is under stress, the need is even greater. That's when good nutrition acts as a backup, a fresh reserve that repeatedly lends support and promotes healing.

Good nutrition starts with maintaining a balanced diet. Addressing specific skin challenges may require emphasizing particular nutrients and making dietary adaptations. A basic balanced diet is what you want to start with if you want optimal health for your skin and the rest of your body.

We are constantly inundated with all sorts of nutritional advice and claims about the latest dietary fads. The best advice is to avoid the fads and build a balanced diet that is designed for your specific needs. A balanced diet has the following components:

- It's nutritious.
- It's portion-controlled (and thus calorie-controlled).
- It's balanced among complex carbohydrates (most containing fiber), lean proteins, and high-quality fats (primarily heart-healthy, skin-healthy unsaturated fats).
- It's made up mostly of whole, unprocessed foods.
- It's plant-based—more vegetables, whole grains, and fruits and less meat.
- It's anti-inflammatory.
- It contains minimal if any amounts of processed foods and nutrient-void ingredients (empty calories).
- It's consumed throughout the day in three meals and two or three snacks.
- It's delicious!

Even in a balanced diet, it's not the foods themselves that directly affect your skin (unless you're applying a homemade egg or honey mask, of course—which is also good!). It's the nutrients in the foods, once metabolized, that make their way to your skin to protect, repair, rebuild, and replenish its needs. When we are pregnant, under stress, going through menopause, or treating a serious illness, our bodies send nutrients to repair and protect our skin. A consistently nutritious diet is even more imperative at these times.

To a significant degree, your diet is one of the few things you can control when everything else is out of control. I can promise you that the good nutritional choices you make to speed healing or the demands of changing hormones will make it easier to adopt healthy eating habits for the rest of your life.

Know Your Nutrients

When you're dealing with skin challenges and the underlying issues that have caused them, you will receive a lot of advice about nutrients and dietary supplements. Although this advice is always well-meaning, too much of what is said usually focuses on the latest trend or "miracle" supplement.

Nutrients have a vital role in the foods that form the backbone of a good balanced diet. We're designed to be resilient and powerful human beings who can receive the nutrients we need from the foods we consume. You cannot replace all those nutrients by taking supplements. They will never make up for a poor diet. Supplements are designed for specific conditions (such as pregnancy), and you should always consult with your health care professional before embarking on a supplement program.

Choose locally grown foods that are organic (pesticide-free) whenever possible. Every day, aim to eat a purer whole-foods diet. The bonus is nutritional synergy. When you eat a whole-foods diet that is plant-based, you experience a synergy from the naturally occurring compounds in the foods themselves. They work with other food components, like natural fiber and phytonutrients (the active compounds in plants), to boost your immune response and overall health. You can't get this from supplements alone.

Vitamins, minerals, antioxidants, proteins, healthy fats, and water all play a significant role in the health and resilience of your skin. Yet even though specific nutrients are vital to healthy skin and overall wellness, nutrients themselves are not enough. It takes a constant, regular, delicious input of nutritious and skin-healthy food to reap the benefits of good energy, vibrant skin, and good overall health.

Superskin Foods: What to Eat to Get the Best Skin Ever

You may have heard the term *superfoods* before. These are foods that have been shown, through multiple well-designed scientific studies, to enhance and protect our health and reduce the risk of chronic diseases. However, these foods have to be more than just scientifically sound. They have to be available to us at any grocery store, they have to be easy to incorporate into our meals throughout the day, and they have to taste great.

Just knowing that a food is a superfood is hardly enough—you have to be able to *eat* it. Availability, versatility, and flavor are the keys. Since the concept of superfoods was introduced, these foods continue to impress researchers and everyday eaters with their ability to help us feel healthy, energized, and at our metabolic, vital best.

Superfoods are health-promoting, disease-fighting foods that are easy to find, easy to use, versatile, and tasty to enjoy on your plate every day. Eating more superfoods as part of your balanced diet ensures that you're getting enough nutrients (vitamins, minerals, fiber, phytonutrients, and potent antioxidants) to keep your immune system boosted and your overall health, including your skin, at its best.

Superfoods, Superspices, and Their Sidekicks

- Avocado
- Beans: all dried beans (such as black beans, kidney, pinto, navy great northern white, garbanzo, lentils), plus string beans, sugar snap peas, green peas, and canned low-sodium beans
- Berries: purple grapes, cranberries, boysenberries, raspberries, straw-

berries, fresh currants, blackberries, cherries, and all other varieties of fresh or frozen berries
- Citrus: oranges, lemons, white and pink grapefruit, kumquats, tangerines, limes
- Dark chocolate
- Dried Superfruits: cherries, raisins, blueberries, prunes, apricots, cranberries, currants, figs
- Extra-virgin olive oil
- Fruits: apples, pears, plums, kiwi, pineapple, guava, red-fleshed papaya, pomegranates, watermelon, pink grapefruit, strawberry guava, Japanese persimmons
- Grains: oats, wheat germ, ground flaxseed, brown rice, barley, wheat, buckwheat, rye, millet, triticale, bulgur wheat, amaranth, quinoa, kamut, yellow corn, wild rice, spelt, whole-wheat couscous
- Honey
- Nuts/Seeds: Walnuts, almonds, pistachios, pumpkin and sunflower seeds, macadamia nuts, pecans, hazelnuts, cashews, Brazil nuts, peanuts (yes, "technically" a legume)
- Poultry: turkey, skinless chicken breast
- Seafood: wild salmon, chunk light tuna, sardines, herring, trout, bass, oysters, clams
- Soy: tofu, soy milk, soy nuts, edamame, tempeh, miso
- Superspices: cinnamon, cumin, oregano, thyme, turmeric, red pepper, ginger, rosemary, black pepper, cloves
- Tea: green and black
- Tomatoes
- Vegetables: broccoli, Brussels sprouts, cabbage, kale, turnips, cauliflower, collard greens, bok choy, mustard greens, swiss chard, pumpkin, carrots, butternut squash, sweet potato, spinach, orange bell pepper, onions, garlic, shallots, leeks, chives
- Yogurt and kefir

Just as superfoods are the key to complete nutrition, many of the superfoods and others I've identified with special properties related to healthy skin also boost your skin's overall vibrancy, resilience, and healthiness.

Dr. Ava affectionately calls them "superskin foods." Certain foods stand out when it comes to skin as great sources of antioxidants, which stop free radicals from damaging collagen, elastin, and skin cells. Still others provide key nutrients, like protein, biotin, and lutein, which are essential for good skin health.

Superskin Foods

Almonds are a friend to the skin on many levels. They are an excellent source of vitamin E, an important antioxidant that protects the skin from photodamage, and a contributor to healthy cell structure and cell tissue. Almonds provide healthy unsaturated fats, which are good for heart protection and cholesterol regulation and which provide an essential part of the cellular membrane on each of the body's cells, including every skin cell. Almonds are an excellent source of the skin-healthy B vitamin biotin. Almonds, as well as other nuts, are a healthy part of a weight-balanced diet. They help with satiety, the sense of feeling satisfied before we're too full.

Avocados are another source of biotin, and they also contain heart- and skin-healthy monounsaturated fats (MUFAs), which provide the ceramides that are important in creating healthy skin cells. MUFAs contribute to skin's natural oil barrier and may reduce dryness. While you're eating an avocado, you might want to moisturize with it, too! There are an increasing number of recipes that incorporate avocado into a luxurious homemade skin care treatment. (See chapter 11 for how to incorporate avocado into your homemade facials and masks.)

Beans also contain biotin, which is the most important B vitamin for your skin. Biotin plays a role in forming skin, hair, and nails, all important components of a healthy appearance. Lentils, kidney beans, soybeans, and peanuts are top-notch sources of biotin.

Blueberries are an excellent source of vitamin C, which is necessary for the production of collagen. The red-blue pigment found in blueberries is a powerful antioxidant that supports the structure of the skin.

Eggs, according to recent research, may contain more bioavailable lutein (an antioxidant that helps skin to maintain its useful appearance) than green vegetables. Eggs are also a great source of protein, which builds the muscles and the tissue below the skin that support its outward appearance. Check with your health care professional for advice on eggs if you have an issue with cholesterol.

Green tea is a rich source of polyphenols and other antioxidants that defend the body and the skin from pollution, the daily effects of living, and cell turnover. Polyphenols also act as an anti-inflammatory and protect the skin from the effects of UVB damage. Green tea may boost metabolism.

Salmon, sardines, and mackerel contain essential fatty acids (EFAs), especially omega-3, which protect the heart and the brain. Omega-3 also has an anti-inflammatory effect on the skin. Salmon also contains a carotenoid called astaxanthin, which helps preserve skin elasticity. Because wild salmon contains high concentrations of anti-inflammatories, it can reduce the symptoms and occurrence of inflammatory skin conditions that cause redness and swelling, like acne, rosacea, and certain rashes. (Always choose wild salmon; farm-raised fish may contain a higher level of toxins.)

Tomatoes contain a number of nutrients, like vitamin C and lycopene, a powerful carotenoid that protects the skin. The carotenoids and other compounds in tomatoes are potent antioxidants that reduce production of free radicals. Eating cooked tomatoes and tomato products like tomato sauces and pastes regularly helps to keep the skin's defenses at their fighting best. Watermelon, pink grapefruit, and strawberry guava also contain lycopene.

Vitamin C–rich foods nourish the skin. Some excellent sources are kiwi, oranges, red and green bell peppers, grapefruit, vegetable and tomato juice, strawberries, broccoli, cantaloupe, pineapple, and mango. Vitamin C deficiencies contribute to dry skin, easy bruising, and reduced elasticity. They can also make it more difficult for the skin to heal. Because of vitamin C's important role in promoting healthy skin, it is also a common ingredient in topical skin care products.

Yellow curry   Many herbs and spices are potent sources of natural antioxidants and act as anti–inflammatories, but research suggests that turmeric, the golden spice that gives yellow curry its color, may reduce the risk of certain skin diseases. A 2009 study demonstrated that curcumin and galangal (a spice in the ginger family) also offered strong protection from UV damage. Although it's still too early to be conclusive, other studies have shown that the active compound in turmeric exhibits strong antioxidant, anti-inflammatory, and anti-tumor properties.

Examples of how to incorporate superskin foods into your meal plan can be found at the end of this chapter.

Using Nutrition to Fight Inflammation

One of the most important skin-healing skills you can learn is how to use good nutrition to fight inflammation.

You're already familiar with inflammation. If you get a scratch or a cut, you may experience pain, tenderness, swelling, and/or redness in the affected area. Inflammation occurs inside the body, too—in the blood vessels, the joints, and even in and around our cells. Chronic inflammation in the body can increase our risk for heart disease, joint problems, and skin complications.

Many skin conditions are either triggered or worsened by inflammation. The body's natural response to assault, inflammation, literally turns up the heat. It revs up your metabolism, churns out cortisol (the stress hormone), and pumps up body temperature. Just as with any immune response, inflammation is intended to be self-limiting. The fever burns out the infection, sweat clears toxins from the pores, and the stress subsides. However, inflammation leaves behind harmful debris in the form of free radicals and other by-products that damage cells and cause other lingering effects.

Dealing with external inflammation is simple: you keep the bump or the scratch clean as it heals, and you try not to hit the same area again. When you're dealing with inflammation inside the body, the best "cure" involves what you eat and how you live.

The Anti-Inflammatory Diet Basics

There are certain foods that appear to increase inflammation and others that have a strong anti-inflammatory effect. Since many skin conditions are inflammatory by nature, decreasing inflammation in the body promotes optimal skin health.

When you follow an anti-inflammatory diet, you work to achieve three goals:

1. Eat in moderation to maintain a healthy weight.
2. Decrease the consumption of foods that increase inflammation.
3. Add foods that can cool or decrease inflammation.

An anti-inflammatory diet does not exclude any food group. Rather, it features the best of the best from all the major food groups, including wholesome carbohydrates and fiber, lean proteins, healthy fats, and low-sugar, high-nutrient, water-filled beverages. Here are some examples:

Carbohydrates   Whole grains—quinoa, brown rice, whole-grain pasta, and whole-wheat bread, cereals, and crackers—can help to manage inflammation through their nutrients, energy, and high-fiber values. Moderation is the key. Fruits and vegetables are also a healthy source of carbohydrates. They are high in water, antioxidants, vitamins, minerals, and fiber and have a strong anti-inflammatory effect on the body, along with many other health benefits. Eating a lot of fresh fruits and vegetables is essential in an anti-inflammatory diet.

Proteins   High-fat proteins, especially meats that are high in saturated fat, increase inflammation. If you don't practice strict portion control, whole-fat dairy and high-fat cheeses can increase inflammation. In contrast, lean proteins (lean poultry, fish, beans, and moderate portions of nuts and seeds) can cool the fire of inflammation.

Fats and oils   Saturated fats, trans fats (hydrogenated oils, found mostly in processed foods like baked goods), and fried foods increase inflammation. Meat, butter, cheese, and other whole-fat dairy products are high in saturated fats. Commercial packaged baked goods like doughnuts, cookies, and cakes often have high levels of saturated and trans fats—a recipe for inflammatory disaster. Liquid oils—like olive oil, canola oil, walnut oil, and other nut oils—can reduce inflammation when used and consumed in moderation. The best anti-inflammatory fats are essential fatty acids, like omega-3 and omega-6. Particularly useful are the omega-3 fatty acids found in salmon, sardines, walnuts, and ground flaxseed and the other polyunsaturated and monounsaturated oils, found in olive oil, olives, avocado, nuts, and seeds.

Beverages   High-nutrient, low-sugar beverages can aid in reducing inflammation. Your body, especially your skin, needs plenty of water. Plain or bubbly water, low-sodium vegetable juices and broths, soups, and low-fat or fat-free milk help with hydration and provide quality nutrition in an anti-inflammatory, skin-boosting diet. Fruits and vegetables can supply up to 20 percent of your water needs, and you should incorporate them as part of a balanced diet every day.

Pro-Inflammatory Foods to Limit or Avoid

- Barbecue sauce and other sugary marinades and sauces
- Bread, bagels, pita, rolls, and tortillas made with refined enriched white flour
- Candy
- Cakes
- Cheese: most varieties, but especially hard cheeses
- Cookies
- Corn syrup, high-fructose corn syrup (check labels carefully)
- Fried foods of all kinds
- Full-fat dairy: butter, cream, half-and-half, ice cream, whole milk, yogurt
- Hydrogenated oils (trans fats): found mostly in packaged baked goods
- Jellies, jams, and preserves, especially if sugar is the first ingredient listed
- Nondairy creamers (they're made from hydrogenated oils and corn syrup)
- Pastries, croissants, and doughnuts
- Processed meats: hot dogs, sausage, bologna, bacon
- Red meat with heavy marbling
- Store-bought muffins and pies
- Sodas (avoid sugary sodas and limit diet sodas to occasional consumption, if any)
- Sugary drinks: fruit drinks, bottled sweetened teas, sweetened coffee beverages, or fruit juices sweetened with added sugar or corn syrup
- Sugar: any kind
- Sweetened cereals (with more than 10 grams sugar per serving)

Anti-Inflammatory Foods That Keep Your Skin Healthy and Clear

- Apples
- Avocados
- Blueberries
- Broccoli
- Cantaloupe
- Cauliflower
- Cherries
- Cinnamon
- Colorful fruits and vegetables
- Ginger and galangal
- Ground flaxseed
- Kiwi
- Mushrooms
- Nuts of all kinds
- Oats
- Olive oil
- Oranges
- Peanuts
- Lean proteins like turkey, chicken breast, egg whites, low-fat or fat-free dairy, soy, lentils, and other beans
- Red pepper (cayenne or paprika)
- Rosemary
- Salmon (wild), sardines, mackerel, and other cold-water fatty fish
- Seeds, especially pumpkin seeds
- Spinach, romaine lettuce, and dark leafy greens
- Tomatoes
- Turmeric (yellow curry)

How to Eat to Fight Inflammation

Incorporate these anti-inflammatory eating habits into your life for clear, healthy skin at all times:

- **Drink water, water, everywhere.** Water hydrates, helping to flush out toxins and keep metabolic levels in balance. From the inside out, nothing beats water. Drink at least eight to ten cups a day—spread throughout the day, not gulped at one time. Drink more if you're active.
- **Harness the power of green tea.** Hot or iced, green tea adds powerful antioxidants to the hydrating value of water. If you absolutely must sweeten your tea, use just a little honey (measure it, to be sure).
- **Eat more fruits and vegetables.** You can accomplish this by eating at least one fruit or vegetable at every meal.
- **Have a vegetable-based soup or garden salad every day.**
- **Choose high-quality, lean proteins.** This will balance your energy and glycemic response.

Are there any foods that I can eat to help my skin as it struggles with acne? Menopausal symptoms? Cancer treatments?

It is important to incorporate a variety of superskin and anti-inflammatory foods into your daily menu for optimal skin health. Here are some suggested foods for combatting health challenges:

- **Acne**   couscous, eggplant, fish oil, onions, ginger, grapefruit, lemons, limes, quinoa, raspberries, sage
- **Cancer**   beans, berries, broccoli, cauliflower, cabbage, kale, dark green leafy vegetables, flaxseed, garlic, onions, scallions, leeks, chives, grapes, green tea (decaf), soy, tomatoes, whole grains
- **Menopause**   dandelion greens, grapefruit, kamut, tempeh, seaweed, avocados, dried plums, chia seeds, beets, pumpkin, edamame, soy nuts, walnuts, tofu, soy milk

- **Go low-fat.** Consume low-fat or even fat-free milk or yogurt in place of full-fat (whole) varieties.
- **Fish for omega-3.** Consume fish that is rich in omega-3s at least two to three times a week or take a daily fish oil supplement.
- **Go nuts.** Enjoy a handful of nuts (about twenty-three almonds, fourteen walnuts, or forty-nine pistachios) per day.
- **Use healthy oils.** Use extra-virgin olive oil, grape seed oil, flaxseed oil, walnut oil, and avocado oil exclusively and sparingly. Eliminate the use of corn oil, safflower oil, and sunflower oil.
- **Spice it up.** Sprinkle in anti-inflammatory, flavorful herbs and spices instead of salt, sugar, and fat. Use herb- and spice-based oil and citrus marinades instead of barbecue sauce, which can be high in sugar.
- **Play fair with portions.** Avoid eating *too much* food—over the course of the day and at one time (meal or snack.)
- **Eat clean.** This means eating mostly whole foods, organically and/or locally grown (if you can find them), and far fewer processed foods.

Putting It All Together: How to Eat for Healthier Skin

How you eat can often be just as important as what you eat. So it's time not only to add more superskin foods into your diet but also to address some of your other bad eating habits. The amazing thing is that even though it may take a bit of time for dietary changes to show up as better cholesterol or blood pressure numbers, the effect on your skin can start happening in one to two days.

Observe What You Eat

An especially good way to inaugurate a better nutritional lifestyle is to begin keeping a food diary. Don't worry—this is not the dreaded calorie counter and fat gram log you may have kept in the past when you tried to drop fifteen pounds in one week. The goal of this food diary is not to judge but to observe. It's important to be candid about your choices. The only person who will see this diary is you, and there's no point in lying to yourself. To start:

1. Get a notebook or a journal—one you like writing in.
2. Pick an area you'd like to learn more about in terms of how your nutritional choices might be affecting you—for example, acne flares, hot flashes, or flagging energy levels.
3. Start keeping track of what you eat. For each meal, include the following information: the date, which meal it is, the time you ate, the various foods that made up the meal, and the approximate portion sizes of each.
4. Make note of what you eat and drink (including water) between meals.
5. To provide more context, you can include notes on your moods, the events of the day, the setting for your meals (at home? in a restaurant? on the go? in the hospital?), the level at which you're exercising—anything that plays into your nutritional choices.
6. Track how your nutritional choices and behaviors affect the areas you're concerned about. Over time, the connections will become clearer. You'll begin to see what works for you nutritionally and what doesn't, so subsequent choices will become easier to make.

Since your skin is as unique to you as your fingerprints, keeping this kind of food diary can help you to identify the foods and behaviors that support and enhance your skin's appearance. It will also reveal the triggers that make it worse. It can be incredibly empowering!

Quantity Matters to Your Skin Health

Now that you know about superfoods, the superskin foods, and anti-inflammatory foods (notice how they overlap, making them easier to incorporate), it's time to start considering how much you eat. Obviously, the amount you eat affects your weight, your health, and your skin. It's all about portion control.

Don't frown as you read those words! Portion control does not mean deprivation. It means getting to know the amount of food that is right for you and for your needs. Think of it this way: You walk into a department store and fall in love with a pair of pants you see on a mannequin. You might ask the sales associate where you can find the pants, but it's highly unlikely that you will buy them without at least checking to see if they're available in your size. Better yet, you'll probably want to try them on to make sure that they fit and look good on you.

The same principle applies to the foods you eat, although you probably act very differently at times. You go into a restaurant and order something straight off the menu—especially if it's a healthy menu full of anti-inflammatory foods. Maybe you choose grilled salmon with broccoli and brown rice. When the dish is brought to you, you eat the whole plateful. If you leave any, you feel as though you're dieting, wasting food, or, worse yet, punishing and depriving yourself. But none of this is true. When the meal arrives, it's sized to a generic patron. You are eating a portion that has more than likely been designed to satisfy a bodybuilder, rather than you as an individual.

There are lots of resources available to you for counting calories (books and websites), managing points in the company of others (Weight Watchers), or simply visualizing and using simple portion size guidelines (*The SuperFoodsRx Diet*). Eating for your particular body size, metabolism, and activity level is the sophisticated and energizing way to go.

I recommend using a tennis ball and deck of cards as a way to gauge portion size. Here's how it works.

Deck of Cards

Lean meat, fish, or poultry: approximately three ounces. Most people need about a deck of cards per meal (three to five ounces, depending on metabolism, gender, and activity level).

Tennis Ball

Grains: one-half to two-thirds of a cup of grains or eighty to one hundred calories of bread, rice, cereal, pasta, corn, and starches like potatoes and yams. Most women need about three to four servings (tennis balls) per day, and most men about four to six.

Fruits and vegetables: about half a cup of fruits or vegetables or one cup of leafy greens like spinach and lettuce. Most men and women need five to nine servings (tennis balls) per day. Nine would be a good goal over time, because it may reduce the risk of heart disease. Nine servings is about two cups of fruit and two and a half to three cups of vegetables.

Portion control takes practice—and more practice. But the payoffs for your energy, your waistline, and your healthier skin are worth the effort. Here are some top tips for eating moderately and consistently at every meal:

- **Get a game plan.** Will you order two appetizers, share an entrée, or box up half to take home? It's your choice—but make a plan before you sit down to eat at a restaurant.
- **Balance your diet by balancing your plate.** Use a smaller dinner plate (such as a luncheon plate). Split the plate into one-fourth protein, one-fourth grains, and one-half vegetables and/or fruit.
- **Eat for your size by knowing your serving sizes.** One serving of protein should be no larger than the palm of your hand. A serving of grains (one-half to two-thirds of a cup) should make a mound about the size of a tennis ball. The rest of your plate should be filled with vegetables and/or fruit.
- **Don't bite off more than you can chew.** Put smaller-than-usual bites on your fork or spoon and chew your food thoroughly. Shoot for about fifteen chews per bite. Who's counting? You are!
- **Take a three- to five-minute break after every ten minutes of eating.** Evaluate your appetite. If you're no longer hungry after a break, don't start eating again. The goal is to eat until you're no longer hungry, not until you're full. The feeling of fullness is actually your body signaling discomfort at having too much food to digest at one time.

A Diet Plan to Take Your Skin from Tired to Terrific

Here are four days' worth of menus to get you started on your skin-boosting diet. The menus show you how to incorporate anti-inflammatory nutrients and foods into meals that you'll enjoy. You can follow these directly or interpret them to fit your own eating needs. The point is to look for opportunities to add skin- and other health-promoting foods into your day. Keep in mind that portion control is important, but you should not skip meals. You need three meals and two or three well-planned snacks every day to give you the energy and the nutrition you need to heal and protect your skin for today and for the long run.

Day 1

Breakfast
Omelet with green and red peppers
Side of fresh blueberries
Cup of coffee

Midmorning Snack
Small handful of almonds and raisins
Cup of green tea

Lunch
Whole-grain pita with chicken salad (made with Greek yogurt, mustard, and yellow curry) with romaine lettuce and sliced tomato.
Cup of lentil soup
Sparkling water with a splash of 100 percent grape juice

Afternoon Snack
Whole-grain crackers
¼ cup guacamole
Cup of herbal tea

Dinner
Small spinach salad with mandarin oranges
Baked salmon with orange and thyme relish
Sautéed broccoli
Baked potato with chives

Day 2

Breakfast
Yogurt and fresh berries with a sprinkle of granola or Kashi cereal
Cup of green tea

Midmorning Snack	Piece of fruit or cup of low-sodium vegetable juice
Lunch	Whole-grain tortilla wrap with tuna salad (made with Greek yogurt, chopped celery and apple), sliced tomato, and lettuce
	Cup of vegetable soup
	Iced green tea or water with lemon
Afternoon Snack	Small yogurt with blueberries
	Cup of herbal tea or water with orange slices
Dinner	Extra-lean turkey burger (or vegetable burger) with tomato, lettuce, and whole-grain bun or dinner roll
	Small salad with spinach, tomatoes, cucumbers, and grated carrot
	Baked sweet potato "fries"

Day 3

Breakfast	Oatmeal with almonds, raisins, and milk
	Cup of green tea
Midmorning Snack	Piece of fruit or cup of low-sodium vegetable juice
Lunch	Entrée salad with grilled chicken, vegetables, olive oil and vinegar, or another all-natural dressing
	Side of whole-grain toast
Afternoon Snack	2 tablespoons walnuts and 2 tablespoons dried cherries
	Glass of water with lemon
Dinner	Grilled chicken with rosemary herb rub
	Green beans
	Brown rice
	Berries

Day 4

Breakfast	16-ounce smoothie with banana, fresh or frozen blueberries and strawberries, 2 teaspoons ground flaxseed, yogurt or milk, and 1 scoop whey or soy protein powder
Midmorning Snack	Sliced apple with 1 tablespoon peanut or almond butter
	Cup of green tea

Lunch	Whole-grain pita sandwich with tuna salad (made with Greek yogurt, chopped celery and apple), sliced tomato, and lettuce Cup of vegetable soup
Afternoon Snack	½ cup hummus 1 cup assorted vegetables (carrot sticks, red bell pepper, celery sticks, broccoli florets, cherry tomatoes) Cup of herbal tea or water with orange slices
Dinner	Whole-grain pasta with turkey Bolognese sauce, sprinkled with oregano Side salad of spinach, sliced almonds, mandarin oranges, and a light vinaigrette

Conclusion

A diet replete with antioxidants and anti-inflammatory foods—super-foods and superskin foods—ultimately goes hand in hand with an overall program to support, replenish, and heal your skin. The optimal approach is to integrate dermatological treatments at home and with your health care team, great nutrition that optimizes your skin's vibrant, dynamic health, and an exercise routine that helps your circulation and enhances healing and repair. You can see and feel the benefits: beautiful skin and sparkling energy.

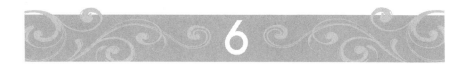

Pregnancy

HOW TO KEEP THE GLOW

A slight, charming thirty-three-year-old actress known for her perfect alabaster skin walked into my office, looking puzzled. "Look," she said, pointing to her face. "This has never happened to me before. I'm tanning, but it's just around my eyes and upper lip!"

"Have you been doing anything different lately?" I asked.

"No!" she said adamantly. "I'm hardly ever in the sun."

I examined her more closely, reached into a drawer, and handed her a pregnancy test. She seemed even more puzzled but said nothing as she headed into the bathroom. Two minutes later, she emerged—in a state of combined panic and elation. The test was positive! She'd had no morning sickness, she told me, and thought nothing of missing a period or two; such a thing is common for a woman who is considered "normal" weight by Hollywood standards but underweight by every other standard.

69

So, how did I know? Her skin. She had melasma, the "mask of pregnancy": light but noticeable blotches of color on her face, as if she had brushed on contouring makeup in all the wrong places. Something about being pregnant makes some women more sensitive to sunlight. The skin darkens, often unevenly.

Motherhood. *Welcome to the first of many startling moments*, I thought.

The old wives' tales about skin during pregnancy are many and contradictory. Before ultrasound, pregnant women thought that they could determine the sex of a child by looking at the condition of their skin, but the skin's appearance really has nothing to do with the gender of a baby.

It's all about hormones. Your new hormonal profile can make your skin significantly better—or frustratingly worse. Indeed, pregnancy's effect on the skin is a little like the weather: given the changes in significant factors (hormonal balance, blood supply, and cell growth), it is absolutely certain that something will happen—but it's impossible to predict exactly what.

When you're pregnant, you may have the most gorgeous complexion you've ever had in your life—the so-called pregnancy glow. This is because your body produces about 50 percent more blood, and that blood carries more oxygen to the skin's surface, causing your face to look brighter. For women who normally have dry skin, extra oil secreted by the sebum glands can add to the dewiness. (Too dewy? That's what a cleanser is for.)

You may also have acne like never before, plus all sorts of annoying little skin problems. Pregnancy is a special state: you are responsible not only for yourself but also for your developing fetus. In the same way that you use extra caution about what you eat and drink, you also need to find safe skin solutions during this period, because when your baby is growing inside you, that's what you want your body to be concentrating on. You don't want to overload it with any unnecessary chemicals or treatments. Once the baby is born, there are many things you can do to solve any skin issues that have cropped up during the nine months. While you are pregnant, there are many skin care products that are safe to use for you and your growing baby.

Over the course of the pregnancy, enormous hormonal shifts occur. The ratio of estrogen to progesterone shifts significantly, with both hormones rising dramatically throughout the pregnancy and estrogen far outpacing progesterone. Because these hormonal changes occur in steps, you may have an issue in your first trimester, such as acne, that may be completely gone by your second trimester. A totally new skin issue, such as stretch marks, may make its first appearance in late pregnancy.

In this chapter you will learn:

- How pregnancy affects your skin
- How to heal your skin: The Dr. Ava Plan
- Postpregnancy rejuvenation options
- Nutrition and fitness tips for better-looking skin
- Skin care regimens during pregnancy

The Impact of Pregnancy on Your Skin

Here are some of the most common skin problems of pregnancy—and what, if anything, you can do about them while the baby is developing.

Acne Breakouts

If acne has been a problem in your life in the past, it may now come back (though probably not with the severity of adolescence). If it hasn't been a problem before, acne may make an unwelcome appearance now because of your pregnancy-level hormones. Acne tends to occur during the first trimester and usually resolves on its own as your estrogen level rises. It may appear in areas where you never experienced acne before, such as your neck, jawline, cheeks, and back. It can be cystic and painful, or your skin can be studded with miniature comedones that look like pebbles on a beach.

In a small percentage of pregnant women, acne in all forms can persist throughout the entire pregnancy. This tends to be the case in women who have a history of severe teenage acne and is most likely related to the elevation of progesterone that occurs during pregnancy.

What to do: Different rules apply to skin care during pregnancy due to the unknown effect that even acne creams may have on a developing baby. All oral acne medications must be avoided. Even some of the most common topical treatments for acne are dangerous now and during breast-feeding. This includes most anti-acne agents such as salicylic acid and retinoids—either over-the-counter retinol or prescription forms like Retin-A and benzoyl peroxide. However, glycolic acid, a commonly used over-the-counter product for acne, is safe to use at this time.

General Principles

- Use a gentle cleanser. Even though your skin is breaking out, it is more sensitive due to the pregnancy and more likely to develop discoloration after the acne is resolved. Anything that is too harsh will only increase the risk of excess pigmentation. Use nonsulfate, nondetergent cleansers.
- Check with your physician about any acne product that you want to use during pregnancy, including spot treatments.
- Exercise caution with all over-the-counter acne procedures, such as home microdermabrasion or home peels.
- Be careful with "natural" ingredients, especially aromatherapy ingredients. Your skin is more sensitive to developing an allergic reaction to them.
- If you suffer from morning sickness, look for fragrance-free treatments. Many otherwise wonderful aromas like rosemary or lavender can make you queasy.
- Don't pick at, pop, or otherwise attempt any do-it-yourself acne "surgery" at home. You risk not only giving yourself a permanent scar but also creating an open wound that can then become infected. This is especially true if you have a toddler in diapers, if you have pets, or if you work outside the home.
- Buy fresh makeup and either clean your makeup brushes or replace all of them. Too much makeup can give you acne instead of covering it up.
- Use water-based or oil-free moisturizers with anti-inflammatory ingredients such as green tea extract, pomegranate, or calendula.
- Use products that have been designed for sensitive skin, because your skin is indeed sensitive during this time. You can also make your own (see chapter 11).

- Instead of sunscreen, use sunblock, which tends to be free of chemicals, or try a sunblock designed for babies. Don't forget to wear a hat, sunglasses, and sunprotective clothing, because UV radiation can not only damage your skin but also worsen your acne.
- Become an amateur scientist. Read labels and know your ingredients.

Assorted Rashes

There are a number of rashes (distinct from acne) that can crop up during pregnancy. For example, if you have a history of eczema and dry, scaly patches of skin that have not appeared for many years, they may return. Otherwise they may occur now for the first time.

There are specific rashes associated with pregnancy. The most common one is pruritic urticarial papules and plaques of pregnancy (PUPPP) and tends to begin on your swollen abdomen in the last six weeks of pregnancy. The rash can range from a few hivelike bumps to red itchy welts that cover your entire torso and extremities.

Another is prurigo of pregnancy, which appears as many tiny bumps that look like bug bites, usually on the hands, feet, arms, and legs, although they can develop anywhere on the body. No one knows what causes it except that it occurs during the final two months of usually a first pregnancy. Although it resolves on its own after the birth of the baby, it can be tricky to manage the itch.

Be sure that you have not developed an allergic reaction to a lotion you are using on your body. These rashes can look identical.

What to do: Although the only cure for the condition is to have the baby, there are a number of ways to try to relieve the itching. These include the following:

- Oatmeal baths
- Calamine lotion
- Nondetergent cleansers or cleansers that double as moisturizers
- Fragrance-free laundry detergent (no dryer sheets)
- Bland moisturizer
- Oral antihistamine (consult your physician first)

Darkening of Moles and Freckles

Increased hormones cause changes in skin pigmentation. You will notice that areas with darker pigmentation, such as freckles, moles, nipples, areolas, and labia, can become even darker.

What to do: If you notice that a mole or a freckle changes in appearance or shape, you should contact your health care provider immediately.

Dry, Itchy Abdomen

For reasons that aren't quite clear, the mother's expanding belly often makes the abdomen skin dry and itchy. The bigger the belly, the worse the itching. One theory is that the stretching of the skin damages the underlying connective tissue, which triggers an inflammatory, allergic-like response.

Annoying as it is, this dryness is very rarely a serious issue. If the itching is accompanied by nausea, vomiting, loss of appetite, fatigue, and possibly yellowing of the skin, then it's time to call your doctor, because it may be a sign of a problem called *cholestasis*. This is a problem not just for the mother but possibly for the developing baby.

What to do: Keep your abdomen moisturized or try a soothing oatmeal bath. You can also try anti-itch creams with topical antihistamines to provide more relief. Try not to scratch; instead, apply a plain, pure aloe vera gel for relief. Even cutting off a piece of an aloe vera plant and applying its juice directly to your abdomen may help. Cool compresses also help. Be sure to limit your time in the bathtub; take a warm, not hot, shower, and always moisturize when you get out of the water. Bubble baths, fragrances, wool, and common allergens such as dust or pet dander can also make you itchy.

Linea Nigra

Linea nigra (Latin for "black line") is the dark vertical line that appears on the abdomen of about 75 percent of all pregnant women in the fourth or fifth month of pregnancy. Like melasma, it's also thought to be caused by increased estrogen. (The line is usually there before pregnancy, but you may not have noticed it until it decided to darken and run like a river down the center of your belly.)

What to do: Nothing, because the line will fade a month or two after the baby is born. If you're wearing something revealing, you may use cover-up.

Melasma

Melasma, the mask of pregnancy, is a brown or tan skin discoloration on the face. It's caused by extra estrogen in the body, which makes pigment cells more sensitive to sunlight.

What to do: Expectant mothers may have to look like Charlie Chaplin for a while, since traditional brightening ingredients like hydroquinone should be avoided during pregnancy. To minimize the darkening, stay out of the sun and be hypervigilant about using a broad-spectrum sunscreen. You might also try a sunscreen moisturizer with a soy blend, like Aveeno Positively Radiant Daily Moisturizer SPF 30, which hydrates well without feeling heavy and may also have some mild lightening effect on the skin. Light diffusers in the formula can also camouflage the pigmentation.

Skin Tags

Skin tags are small, loose growths of skin that usually appear during pregnancy under your arms, on your neck, on your breasts, or even around your groin. If they are irritating to you, they can be removed by a doctor.

What to do: After pregnancy, your skin tags may disappear. If they do not disappear, see your doctor. If they become irritated, apply hydrogen peroxide followed by an antibiotic ointment.

Spider Veins

Spider veins are tiny weblike reddish or bluish veins that branch outward underneath the skin. They may appear not only on the legs but also on the face, neck, chest, and upper arms and are caused by tiny blood vessels dilating with all the additional blood in the body. Spider veins tend to occur during the second and third trimester and are due to increased estrogen.

Red blotches that look like spider veins can occur after vomiting associated with severe morning sickness. These blotches will go away on their own.

What to do: Most of the time, spider veins that developed with pregnancy will disappear several months after pregnancy. If not, wait until after the baby is born to seek further treatment (see the section below on postpregnancy rejuvenation).

Stretch Marks

Stretch marks are exactly what they sound like: visible reddish or purplish lines in the middle layer of skin (the dermis) that can occur when we gain weight rapidly, which stretches the skin. They occur particularly in pregnancy, not only because of the stretching but also because of the increased influx of hormones. Why some women get them but others don't is unknown. When we look at them under the microscope, we see tears in the collagen in the deeper layers of the skin.

Stretch marks also occur during adolescent growth spurts, which makes their cause even more mysterious. They are harmless, if not particularly attractive. If untreated, they will usually fade into a silvery hue.

What to do: Cocoa butter has a reputation for being the go-to stretch-mark-prevention treatment, but there's no evidence that it works. Most creams have a small percentage of cocoa butter, so if you are going to use it, be sure you find one that is 100 percent real cocoa butter. One study found that a daily application of a cream containing gotu kola extract and vitamin E was associated with fewer stretch marks during pregnancy, but the study has not been successfully replicated. Your best chance at prevention is to follow your doctor's guidelines for weight gain.

Varicose Veins

Varicose veins are tubular bluish veins that can appear on the legs during pregnancy. The pressure of the growing baby on the veins deep in your abdomen and the additional blood flow can make your leg veins bulge.

Normally, blood in the body travels in one direction, and little valves in the veins are supposed to keep the blood from going backward. However, with all the extra blood and pressure, sometimes these valves just don't close properly. If this is the case, the blood backs up and pools in the veins, which dilates the vessels and causes swelling in the legs and ankles. Varicose veins usually don't hurt, but they can ache—and they're not exactly a boon to body image when you already feel like a bloated tick.

What to do: To some degree, varicose veins are genetic, so if they run in your family, you may not be able to avoid them entirely. To minimize the symptoms, do the following:

- Walk as much as possible. Walking helps the blood to return to the heart, whereas standing still allows the blood to pool in your legs.
- When you're sitting, prop your feet up—and try not to sit for long periods. If possible, prop your legs higher than your head for half an hour a day.
- Get support stockings. Yes, you might feel like your great-aunt Sadie, but they do help.
- Make sure you get enough vitamin C, which is important for the health and elasticity of your veins. (After pregnancy, regular vitamin C may help the veins bounce back to their normal size and shape.)
- Avoid excessive weight gain. Obviously, the thirty to thirty-five pounds gained in a normal pregnancy will not be as hard on your legs as sixty or sixty-five pounds. (If you're having twins or triplets, ignore this. You should be gaining more weight, depending on the pregnancy.) Always follow guidelines set by your doctor.

After the baby is born, varicose veins may disappear within a few months—unless you had them before the pregnancy, in which case they will probably remain and perhaps get worse. There are various treatments for variscosities that vascular surgeons can perform, including surgery or lasers threaded inside the dilated vein.

Wrinkles

More and more women are putting off pregnancy until later in life. But is it safe to continue an anti-aging skin regimen while pregnant? What can you do to keep your pregnant skin looking young no matter what your age?

What to do: You are certainly entitled to a hydrating or gentle cleansing facial, but any product containing Retin-A must be avoided. Products that contain antioxidants, glycolic acid, or peptides are generally safe, but be sure to check with your health care provider. All forms of skin lighteners, either botanicals (such as kojic acid or licorice extract) or hydroquinone, must be avoided at this time.

Skin Gone Wild

There's an excellent chance that at least one of the conditions above will happen to you when you're pregnant, because they're all annoyingly common manifestations of pregnancy. There are two rarer conditions that are unlikely, but it's useful to be aware of them. Either of the following requires an urgent visit to your doctor:

Pemphigoid gestationis   This is an autoimmune disorder that begins with very itchy red hives or bumps around the belly button, usually in the second or third trimester. The rash usually spreads to form circular patterns on the skin and can appear just about anywhere on the body (but usually not the face or the scalp). After a couple of weeks, blisters form, and if they are not infected, they'll heal without scarring. This rash can affect the health of the baby and should be addressed immediately. The presence of this rash may indicate a problem with the pregnancy and should be brought to the attention of your general practitioner.

Pustular psoriasis of pregnancy   This is very rare and little understood. People who have pustular psoriasis (they usually do not suffer from the more common, itchy-red-patch form of psoriasis) have clearly defined, raised bumps on the skin that are filled with pus.

Large portions of your skin may redden; even worse, you may also experience vomiting, diarrhea, fever, and chills. The condition is quite serious and requires immediate attention from your doctor.

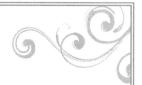

Pregnancy Skin Care
A CASE STUDY

"No Pictures, Please"

Patient: Terry, Asian, mid-thirties

Everyone always talks about the pregnancy "glow." However, the hormones associated with Terry's four-month-old pregnancy caused her once-perfect skin to break out in cystic acne and comedones.

"I was so looking forward to being pregnant," she said when she came to see me. "I even wanted my husband to take lots of pictures to show how my body changed with each trimester. Now I can't even stand to look at myself in the mirror."

The cysts were painful, and she wasn't sure how she should treat them. Terry had had mild acne as a teenager and had used over-the-counter topicals to keep it under control.

"I'm not sure what to do," she said to me. "I hear that most acne prescriptions and over-the-counter stuff are not recommended for pregnant women."

Treatment Plan

Terry was right. Prescription acne medications and even over-the-counter topical anti-acne products can be harmful during pregnancy. To help clear her skin, I recommended a series of safe, deep-cleansing facials. I also adjusted her skin care program to include glycolic acid and products that are oil-free and contain anti-inflammatories, antioxidants, and good UV radiation protection.

When I saw her again a few months later, Terry definitely had the glow. "I can feel the baby moving," she stated happily, "and now that I have my skin under control, I feel beautiful. My husband showers me with compliments about how I look. I tell him, 'Take all the pictures you want!'"

Healing Your Skin: The Dr. Ava Plan

In so many ways, pregnancy is like the great unknown. It is miraculous yet terrifying at the same time. You know that something really wonderful is going on, but you don't know what your body is doing. Your skin is a little perplexed, too: one day it's oily, the next day it's dry. At the beginning of your pregnancy, you might be breaking out like a teenager. At the end of your pregnancy, your skin might be the most beautiful it's ever been in your entire life. Then, after your pregnancy, your skin might dry out.

All of these changes are due to the hormonal curve associated with pregnancy. From the beginning to the end, your estrogen level increases exponentially, thirty to forty times higher than your peak levels during your menstrual cycle. Your progesterone level also rises, not as dramatically, but twenty times higher than your peak levels during your menstrual cycle.

This is why some women continue to break out throughout their entire pregnancies but most women do not. Your skin can change with each trimester, so the recommendations below include ingredients that are considered safe to use throughout pregnancy.

Phase 1: Cleanse and Exfoliate

There is so much going on with your body, and if you also have a toddler pulling at your leg, you may be tempted to neglect your skin. Resist the urge! It's impossible to recommend a definitive skin care program for you, because every individual has unique needs that may change as her pregnancy progresses. Nevertheless, there are some guidelines to follow.

In general, the products you use will need to be different from those in your previous skin regimen. Even though you may not think that your skin is sensitive, the hormonal dance creates sensitive skin. Look for a gentle cleanser that is recommended for sensitive skin. Read the labels and choose a cleanser that is fragrance-free and dye-free and that (ideally) does not include sodium lauryl sulfate.

If you are breaking out, look for a cleanser with glycolic acid; you need to avoid cleansers with salicylic acid and benzoyl peroxide during your pregnancy. Cleansers that contain essential oils may cause an allergic reaction because of your newly sensitive skin. If you have any questions, do a patch test on your arm or your forehead. This is done by taking a small amount of the product and applying it to your skin for about ten minutes. Rinse it off and repeat this process for three days. By doing this, you will know if you are allergic to the product.

Be extremely cautious about exfoliation. Exfoliation may have helped clear your breakouts before pregnancy, but it can aggravate your acne now. The same principle applies to the pregnancy mask, melasma.

This pigmentation cannot be scrubbed off your face, and trying to do so can make it much worse. Avoid using over-the-counter scrubs, and do a patch test with any mechanical exfoliator. The best choice is to use a homemade scrub like baking soda or brown sugar.

Phase 2: Nourish

Your changing body and your developing baby need a special set of nutrients, and so does your skin. You may notice that your hair has never been thicker, your nails have never been stronger, and your skin may have a glow—all of this from the physiology of pregnancy and your prenatal vitamins. During this period, it is important to use products that have real value for your skin. These include antioxidants such as flavonoids (soy extract), polyphenols (pomegranate extract), and carotenoids (papaya). These can be found in many skin care products, but this is a good time to make your own (see chapter 11). Be sure to purchase organically grown fruits.

Phase 3: Moisturize

Once again, your needs may change with each trimester. Choose products that are oil-free and non-comedogenic and that contain calming or soothing ingredients like calendula. Be cautious with ingredients like chamomile or lavender, especially if you have allergies. If your skin is very dry, look for moisturizers that are creamy and that contain emollients and humectants designed for sensitive and dry skin. (Aveeno and Cetaphil are good brands). If your skin feels oily or if you have breakouts, use moisturizers that are lotions and are oil-free. Your antioxidants may be

---

DR. AVA'S MYTH BREAKER

The myth: If the product says "natural," it must be safe to use during pregnancy.

The truth: In this country, we tend to believe that anything that's natural is good for you—or, at the very least, harmless. That is not necessarily true. It is not always the case that anything chemical is bad and that anything that grows on a tree or comes from a plant is good. Natural ingredients can have real effects, and sometimes those effects are not ideal for a developing baby. Sometimes we don't even know what effects they have on a developing baby, since cosmetic companies do not test their products on pregnant women.

Avoid ingesting or rubbing the following essential oils on yourself during pregnancy (they can cross the placental barrier and may cause uterine contractions): anise, basil, bergamot, birch, carrot, catnip, cinnamon, citronella, clove, fennel, ginger, grapefruit, juniper, lemon, lemongrass, marjoram, myrrh, myrtle, orange, peppermint, ravensara, rosemary, tangerine, and thyme.

included in your moisturizer. (See the skin-care regimen later in this chapter for a list of ingredients that are safe to use during pregnancy.)

Phase 4: Rejuvenate

Due to wonderful scientific advances, women have been able to extend their childbearing years. Thus you may find yourself happily pregnant but with wrinkles. During this time, your rejuvenating choices are limited to using alpha-hydroxy lotions and hydrating facials or products that contain hyaluronic acid. These products are effective as long as you use them on a regular basis. Don't give up, and keep in mind that you will have more options available once the baby is born.

Phase 5: Protect

Because a high estrogen level makes your skin more likely to pigment, UV protection is more important than ever. In addition, the function of your immune system is altered during pregnancy, which makes your skin more susceptible to developing skin cancer. All sunblocks are considered to be safe during pregnancy, but now might be a good time to use one that is chemical-free and designed for sensitive skin or babies. Remember that sunblocks aren't perfect, so using a hat or even an umbrella is advisable to prevent the mask of pregnancy. Make sure you reapply your sunblock throughout the day on all exposed areas of the skin.

Postpregnancy Rejuvenation Options

After the miracle of birth has happened, you may look at yourself in the mirror and wonder, *Will I ever look like my "before baby" self?* It seems hard to believe, but yes, you will. Not only can your figure return to your prepregnancy state; so can your skin. Your tummy, which may seem like it's hanging over your pants, usually tightens up on its own as a result of your very own elastic and collagen fibers.

Many of the other skin changes discussed earlier, such as acne or *linea nigra*, will also go away on their own within a year. Other issues may need intervention to speed up their resolution. These recommendations may not apply to you while you are nursing, but don't worry, you can begin soon after nursing. Nursing itself helps your body to regain its former shape.

Here are some postpregnancy rejuvenation recommendations:

Acne   Once you have given birth, it is safe to get peels and laser treatments. Your doctor may also prescribe azelaic acid or topical antibiotics. (See chapter 8 for more information.)

Dry hands   This may be a new problem that presents itself once the baby is born because of all the hand washing you'll be doing and possibly from the irritation caused by using baby wipes. If so, look for sensitive baby wipes. It's also important to use a nondetergent cleanser for your hands, to rinse off any excess soap, and to apply a moisturizer each time you wash your hands. If your hands start to crack and bleed, you can get a prescription moisturizer from your health care provider.

Dry skin   Hydrating facials can combat the dry skin that may result when your estrogen level drops after childbirth. These facials use natural products to restore moisture. An intensive in-office microdermabrasion followed by an infusion of active nutrients, called SilkPeel or Intraceuticals, can effectively nourish and hydrate the skin.

Facial spider veins   These can be removed or reduced with a vascular laser or with intense pulsed light treatment. Bursts of intense light essentially shrink the veins without damaging the skin. Each vein requires a series of treatments with the laser. There may be redness or swelling, but this generally disappears within a few days.

Fat pockets   After the baby is born, you might find that you are left with a small tummy bulge, which can remain even after your skin has tightened up and you are back at your prepregnancy weight. An external fat-freezing device called Zeltiq is ideal for removing this pocket. If you have only sagging, loose skin, there are several new noninvasive options that include different tissue-tightening radiofrequency devices such as Thermage, Accent, and Affirm.

Hair thinning   During your pregnancy you probably enjoyed a luxuriant mane of hair. Between three and six months after the birth of the baby, you may experience a tremendous hair loss in which your hair seems to be falling out in handfuls. This is called a *telogen effluvium*. It occurs because your hair goes into a resting phase and then falls out all at once, like children bolting out of school when they hear the recess bell. It is important to check with your doctor to make sure you don't have anemia, a thyroid problem, or any other illness. Sometimes using an over-the-counter Rogaine solution and taking a biotin supplement can speed the regrowth.

Keratosis pilaris   This is a condition in which tiny rough bumps appear primarily on the backs of the arms and occasionally on the tops of the legs. Tiny buds of keratin (tissue) form at the tip of the hair follicle, giving your skin a rough, bumpy texture like chicken skin. You may experience this rash for the very first time after the birth of your baby. It is associated with eczema and dry skin. The best treatment is a gentle exfoliation in the shower, with either a handheld brush or an exfoliating cream, followed by a moisturizer with an alpha-hydroxy acid or urea. This condition tends to be ongoing, and although your health care professional may be able to smooth it temporarily with an office treatment, you will need to continue an at-home program to keep your skin as soft as your baby's.

Leg veins   Sclerotherapy is a procedure in which medication is injected into the veins to make them shrink. A new injectable solution called Asclera has proven to be very safe and effective for shrinking and dissolving leg veins. Be sure to find a health care provider who is experienced in this technique. Veins can also be treated with lasers, although sclerotherapy is generally more effective, due to the larger size of the vein. The laser process is noninvasive but more time-consuming: one vein generally requires four to six treatments.

Lentigo   This is the name for the brown spots that may have appeared on your face, chest, and/or hands during your pregnancy. There are many options for treating them, beginning with a prescription-strength fade cream that combines a retinoid with a skin lightener. There are over-the-counter choices as well, which contain botanical ingredients such as licorice root, arbutin, or kojic acid. In-office treatment might require liquid nitrogen or lasers that are targeted to remove the excess pigment in your skin.

Melasma If the mask persists after the baby is born—and it often does—wait at least six months before you step up treatment. Options include a 4 percent prescription-strength lightener like hydroquinone; a 10 percent strong glycolic peel to slough off the outer layer of pigmented cells; or a laser to remove pigment from deeper skin layers.

Stretch marks (striae) Once the baby is born, there are many options for improving stretch marks. The reddish-purple color in stretch marks can be mostly, if not entirely, eliminated with a pulse-dye laser like the Candela Vbeam. When you are finished nursing, you can use a retinoid like Retin-A, Differin, or Tazorac to stimulate the skin to repair itself.

Wrinkles When you return to your prepregnancy weight, wrinkles may appear for the very first time. Sleepless nights with the new baby certainly don't help. The goal is to not only soften the wrinkles but also improve the overall appearance of the skin. In the upper third of the face, most wrinkles are caused by motion (such as frowning). In the lower two-thirds of the face, most wrinkles are caused by volume loss that results from ultraviolet damage or tissue thinning. Motion wrinkles are treated with neuromodulators such as Botox and Dysport. Wrinkles created by volume loss can be treated with injectable fillers such as Radiesse, Juvederm, and Restylane.

An at-home skin care routine is the backbone of any rejuvenation program. Throughout this book, I recommend combinations of active ingredients that will stimulate new collagen growth, increase cell turnover, and add nutrients to the skin.

There are many types of lasers used for rejuvenation. One of the newest (with little downtime) is the Isolaz Profusion system, which treats fine lines and wrinkles as well as textural changes of the skin. It delivers active ingredients noninvasively to a deeper level of the skin and is offered through a dermatologist's office.

Dr. Wendy's Eating Well during Pregnancy

During pregnancy, the human body will do whatever it takes to produce a healthy baby—sometimes even at the expense of the mother's health. As a result, you may experience flagging energy, skin issues, or increased susceptibility to colds. Learning what to eat during this important time can help you to optimally fuel yourself and your growing baby.

Your caloric needs will change depending on your height, weight, and activity level. However, you will not be "eating for two." In fact, you will require far fewer extra calories than you may think. (Actual caloric requirements are covered on page 89.)

It is very important to eat nutritious foods and to make smart choices about the timing, portions, and quality of your meals. The goal is to get more of your fuel from nutrient-rich whole foods. Remember, quality first! If you are not eating a high-quality diet, you may suffer as a result, and your skin is the one place it will show. Nourish your baby *and* yourself with the best nutrition you can, and your skin will glow.

Your diet should be based on the following guidelines:

Protein

Remember that you are building a healthy frame that includes muscles, a skeleton, organs, and all the enzymes and hormones necessary to support the frame's function. This requires protein. In pregnancy, women are advised to get about one gram of protein per kilogram of body weight (1 kilogram equals 2.2 pounds). Since body weight changes during pregnancy, your protein needs will, too. Foods with protein include red meat, poultry, fish, beans, soy, nuts, and seeds. Whole grains and beans form a complete protein.

Carbohydrates

Carbohydrates provide energy to fuel both your body and the baby, so this is no time for a no-carb or low-

---

Sample Calculation: Daily Protein Needs

Laurie W.'s starting weight is 140 pounds (140 ÷ 2.2 = 64 kg).

Her starting protein need is 64 grams of protein per day.

Her third-trimester weight is 170 pounds (170 ÷ 2.2 = 77 kg).

Laurie needs 77 grams of protein per day in her last trimester.

carb diet. Instead, carbs should make up 55 to 60 percent of your total daily calories. Carbohydrates include whole grains such as bread, cereal, pasta, crackers, brown rice, quinoa, and corn, as well as whole fruit. A woman on a diet of two thousand calories a day should be eating 275 to 300 grams of carbohydrates a day. This should include three or four fruit servings (one or two of citrus) and four or five servings of whole grains.

Fat

Healthy sources of fat are essential to the proper growth and development of your baby's body, nervous system, organs, and brain. Fat should make up about 30 percent of your total calories, or approximately 67 grams per day on a 2,000-calorie diet. During pregnancy, do the following:

- Eliminate trans fat (hydrogenated oil) as much as possible.
- Limit saturated fat, including butter and other solid fat like the marbling on meat and whole-fat dairy.
- Focus on healthy sources of fat: avocados, nuts, seeds (flax, pumpkin, and chia), olive oil, and fish oil.

Foods to Avoid

Here are a few reminders about foods and ingredients to limit or avoid during pregnancy:

Alcohol   Avoid during pregnancy.

Caffeine   Limit drastically or eliminate. Science is not conclusive about the effects of caffeine on pregnancy, although strong research suggests that small amounts will not harm a growing fetus. However, it is advisable to work on eliminating caffeine from the diet, keeping in mind that an occasional small source of caffeine (such as in chocolate or decaffeinated teas) will most likely not cause any harm.

Artificial sweeteners and refined and processed foods   Limit as much as possible. Avoid commercial sodas and packaged baked goods. This is a great time to clean up your diet in these areas, for both your baby and your skin!

Bacterial risks   To prevent listeriosis, a bacterium that can be harmful to pregnant women and their babies, avoid unpasteurized milk and soft cheese, raw or undercooked red meat, poultry, fish, and shellfish; and prepared deli meats and hot dogs.

Prenatal Vitamins

Along with a nutrient-dense, calorie-sufficient diet, a prenatal vitamin that includes 600 micrograms of folic acid and occasional other individualized supplements is generally all a woman needs to support proper fetal growth.

The supplements, which should be prescribed only by your doctor, may include the following:

- Calcium, to build strong teeth and bones
- Vitamin C, to promote healthy skin, teeth, gums, and bones and increase iron absorption
- Vitamin A, to form healthy skin, eyesight, and bones
- Vitamin B_6, to form red blood cells and help the body to use protein, carbs, and fat for energy and growth
- Vitamin B_{12}, to form red blood cells and a healthy nervous system
- Folate (folic acid), to build blood and protein and protect from nervous system defects
- Iron, to make healthy red blood cells that deliver oxygen to the fetus as well as to the mother

Other Supplement Use

Self-prescribing during pregnancy can be dangerous, and be aware that *natural* does not necessarily mean safe. Check with your doctor before taking any additional vitamins, minerals, herbs, or other supplements.

Keep in mind that more is not better. Hypervitaminosis (excess vitamins) can be as bad as or even worse than not enough vitamins. Follow the recommendations of your pediatrician, your pediatric dietitian, and other licensed health care providers, who can monitor you and make adjustments according to your needs and the phase of your pregnancy.

Weight Gain during Pregnancy

Of course weight gain occurs during pregnancy, but how much is too much, too little, or just right? In 2009, the Institute of Medicine issued updated recommendations about healthy weight gain during pregnancy.

The Institute of Medicine and the American College of Obstetricians and Gynecologists suggest that pregnant women gain the following:

- 28–40 pounds for underweight women
- 25–35 pounds for normal-weight women
- 15–25 pounds for overweight women
- 11–20 pounds for obese women
- 35–45 pounds for women carrying twins

Although it's true that you will need some extra calories to fuel yourself and stimulate the healthy growth and development of your baby, the old adage that you are eating for two is a bit exaggerated. Actually, it's a lot exaggerated, in most cases. Usually, all that's necessary is to add an average of only one to three hundred extra calories per day—total!

Suppose you need 2,000 calories a day. To meet the growing demands of your baby, you should add the following:

- 50–150 calories per day during the first trimester
- 300 calories per day during the second and third trimesters

One hundred calories is equal to about one of the following:

- 10–13 almonds
- 1 cup of nonfat milk
- 1 slice of whole-grain bread or toast
- 1¼ cup of blueberries
- 2 ounces of fish or poultry
- Less than ½ cup of frozen yogurt

> ### Sample Calculation: Weight Gain Goals
>
> Laurie W. is 5 feet 7 inches, and her prepregnancy weight is 140 pounds.
>
> Goal: 25–35 pounds in weight gain, for a total of 165–175 pounds.
>
> First trimester: 2–4 pounds (average 1 pound per month)
> Second trimester: 10–12 pounds (average 1 pound per week)
> Third trimester: 2–17 pounds (average 1 pound per week)

Three hundred calories is equal to about one of the following;

- Half a sandwich: one slice of bread, 1 tablespoon of peanut butter, and 1 medium banana
- Fruit-flavored yogurt and a small handful of nuts
- ⅓ cup of trail mix (nuts and dried fruit)
- 2 store-bought, packaged cookies
- A smoothie made with 12 ounces of fruit, protein powder, and yogurt

As you can see, it really doesn't take a lot to get in the extra calories. This doesn't mean that you can't treat yourself occasionally or give in to the very real cravings during pregnancy when they occur. Just be aware that a little goes a long way.

Omega-3 for Healthy Skin

For optimal nutrition and healthy skin during pregnancy, omega-3 fats are excellent; they are good for your skin, your heart, and the growing fetus. Walnuts, ground flaxseed, and chia seeds are good plant-based sources of omega-3, whereas fish and shellfish are excellent animal-based sources.

However, when it comes to eating fish during pregnancy, some precautions are necessary. The American College of Obstetricians and Gynecologists and the American Heart Association both suggest that pregnant women may eat *up to* twelve ounces of fish per week. Twelve ounces translates into the following:

- Four meals of three-ounce portions
- Three meals of four-ounce portions
- Two meals of six-ounce portions

Keep in mind that these portions both support your healthy skin and weight and allow a greater frequency of eating fish, if you enjoy it. Here are some other suggestions when adding fish to your diet:

- Go for a variety of fish instead of one kind: shellfish, canned fish (choose light tuna instead of albacore), farm-raised catfish, wild salmon, and smaller ocean fish.
- Choose wild salmon over farmed salmon to reduce the possibility of contamination with PCBs.

- Avoid large fish that may contain traces of mercury, especially shark, swordfish, king mackerel, tilefish, and albacore tuna, and limit the frequency of consuming large tuna (stick with chunk light).
- Eat only cooked fish: broiled, baked, or grilled. Avoid sushi or undercooked (such as rare) fish during pregnancy.

Alisa's Fitness Tips

The American College of Obstetricians and Gynecologists suggests that a pregnant woman can engage in thirty minutes (sometimes more) of moderate exercise on most days of the week, provided that she has permission from her physician to do so. Making exercise a regular habit while pregnant will help you to maintain your overall health and the health of your baby, and it will also allow your postpregnancy physique to bounce back faster. Always stay aware and listen to your body. Never push yourself too hard when exercising. If you are out of breath and are unable to carry on a simple conversation, it is best to *slow down*.

After the first trimester, avoid exercises that cause you to lie on your back (which diminishes blood flow to the uterus). Supporting your rear end with a pillow or a rolled towel will alleviate pressure and compression on the vena cava (the large vein that returns blood to the heart).

During pregnancy you can do the following for exercise:

- Take a short walk or walk in place in between extended phases of stationary exercise (yoga poses or resistance training). This will improve circulation and prevent the dizziness associated with decreased uterine blood flow and blood pooling in the legs.
- Swim moderately for fifteen minutes twice a day. This will combat mood swings, improve your quality of sleep, and reduce fatigue.

After the baby is born, invest in a sturdy maternity bra that offers plenty of support when exercising. The correct fit can improve posture, alleviate back pain, and stave off sagging skin on the chest. Be sure to avoid any heavy lifting during the first two weeks after giving birth.

After pregnancy you can do the following:

- You can reintroduce exercise by walking several days per week for ten to fifteen minutes (with your doctor's approval). Walking aids postpregnancy bowel function, facilitates muscle tone, improves circulation to the skin, and prevents blood clot formation. Always start out slowly and be patient with yourself.

- Later, take a brisk walk or a jog with a jogging stroller (three wheels), which offers your baby a smoother ride during naps. This activity can be performed daily and will boost your metabolism, your health, and your postpregnancy mood.
- Invest in household exercise equipment items such as a treadmill, light handheld weights, or various strengths of resistance bands. Keeping these items close will enable you to sneak in extra exercise time when you can.
- Take a postpregnancy yoga class to help you reduce stress, regulate mood swings, and reduce neck and back pain.

Skin Care Regimens during Pregnancy

OILY SKIN

MORNING REGIMEN

Step	Directions
Cleanse	Wash with a soap-free cleanser that contains polyhydroxy acid (PHA).
Tone	If needed, apply an oil-controlling toner.
Eyes	Gently dot a small amount of cream around the eyes. Choose products with ingredients that address your areas of concern. Vitamin K, caffeine, vitamin C, yarrow, horse chestnut, and gingko biloba address dark circles. Haloxyl, caffeine, vitamin C, cucumber extract, green tea, and aloe vera address puffiness. Hyaluronic acid, silica, soy proteins, acai berry, aloe vera, seaweed extracts, GABA, and argireline address wrinkles, firmness, and elasticity.

Moisturize	Every day:
	    Apply a small amount of a light, oil-free, non-comedogenic moisturizer with antioxidants and vitamins.
	
	If you have additional skin care needs:
	    Choose an oil-free moisturizer with ingredients designed to address your specific skin care issues. Azelaic acid, tea tree oil, and glycolic acid address oil production and

breakouts. Mulberry extract, arbutin, bearberry extract, licorice extract, kojic acid, azelaic acid, and gallic acid address discoloration. Green tea, calendula, cucumber, aloe vera, chamomile, willow herb, perilla leaf extract, evening primrose oil, zinc, mallow, red algae, and silymarin address inflammation and irritation.

Protect	Apply an oil-free, broad-spectrum, and non-comedogenic sunblock *every day*. *Note:* If your moisturizer contains a sunscreen of at least SPF 25 that blocks UVA and UVB rays, you don't need to add extra sunblock.

EVENING REGIMEN

Step	Directions
Cleanse	Wash with a soap-free cleanser.
Tone	If needed, gently wipe your face with toner or spray with facial water.
Eyes	Gently dot a small amount of cream around the eyes. Choose products with ingredients that address your areas of concern. Vitamin K, caffeine, vitamin C, yarrow, horse chestnut, and gingko biloba address dark circles. Haloxyl, caffeine, vitamin C, cucumber extract, green tea, and aloe vera address puffiness. Hyaluronic acid, silica, soy proteins, acai berry, aloe vera, seaweed extracts, GABA, and argireline address wrinkles, firmness, and elasticity.
Moisturize	Every evening: Apply a small amount of moisturizing lotion with antioxidants. If you have additional skin care needs: Choose an oil-free moisturizer with ingredients that address your areas of concern. Azelaic acid, tea tree oil, and glycolic acid address oil production and breakouts. Mulberry extract, arbutin, bearberry extract, licorice extract, kojic acid, azelaic acid, and gallic acid address discoloration. Green tea, calendula, cucumber, aloe vera, chamomile, willow herb, perilla leaf extract, evening primrose oil, zinc, mallow, red algae, and silymarin address inflammation and irritation.

INGREDIENTS TO AVOID

If your skin is excessively oily: Mineral oil, petrolatum, coconut oil

If your skin is highly sensitive: Lactic acid, glycolic acid, alpha-lipoic acid, acetic acid, benzoic acid, cinnamic acid, menthol, parabens, quaternium-15, vitamin C

If you have existing discoloration: Celery extract, lime extract, parsley extract, fig extract, carrot extract, bergamot oil, estradiol, genistein

If your skin is acne-prone: Butyl stearate, cinnamon oil, isostearyl isostearate, cocoa butter, jojoba oil, coconut oil, decyl oleate, myristyl myristate, myristyl propionate, octyl palminate, octyl stearate, peppermint oil, isopropyl stearate, isopropyl isostearate, myristate, palmitate

AT-HOME TREATMENTS

You can purchase over-the-counter masks and exfoliates for oily skin, or you can make your own (see chapter 11).

Masks	You can apply a mask once or twice a week to tighten the pores and temporarily reduce excessive oil production. Masks are also helpful in reducing acne inflammation.
Exfoliation	As long as your skin is relatively calm, you can use a gentle exfoliating scrub once a week. If you are experiencing a flare-up of acne or excessive oil production, do not use any kind of scrub.

IN-OFFICE PROCEDURES

Cleansing facial   Hydrating facial   Microdermabrasion

COMBINATION SKIN

MORNING REGIMEN

Step	Directions
Cleanse	Wash with a gentle soap-free cleanser.
Tone	Gently wipe your face with a hydrating toner or facial water.
Eyes	Gently dot a small amount of cream around the eyes. Choose products with ingredients that address your areas of concern. Vitamin K, caffeine, vitamin C, yarrow, horse chestnut, and gingko biloba address dark circles. Haloxyl, caffeine, vitamin C, cucumber extract, green tea, and aloe vera address puffiness. Hyaluronic acid, silica, soy proteins, acai berry, aloe vera, seaweed extracts, GABA, and argireline address wrinkles, firmness, and elasticity.
Moisturize	Every day: Apply a small amount of moisturizer with antioxidants. If you have additional skin care needs: Choose a moisturizer with ingredients designed to treat your specific skin care issues. Glycolic acid, tea tree oil, and zinc address oil production and breakouts. Hyaluronic acid, ceramide, olive oil, evening primrose oil, borage seed oil, colloidal oatmeal, apricot kernel oil, macadamia nut oil, safflower oil, and jojoba oil address hydration. Mulberry extract, vitamin C, pine bark extract, strawberry begonia, and magnesium ascorbyl phosphate address discoloration. Aloe vera, green tea, calendula, cucumber, chamomile,

willow herb, perilla leaf extract, feverfew, evening primrose oil, red clove, mirabilis, colloidal oatmeal, red algae, and zinc address irritation and inflammation. Azelaic acid, tea tree oil, and zinc address acne flares.

Protect	Apply broad-spectrum sunblock *every day*.
	Note: If your moisturizer contains a sunscreen of at least SPF 25 that blocks UVA and UVB rays, you don't need to add extra sunblock.

EVENING REGIMEN

Step	*Directions*
Cleanse	Wash your face with a cleanser that contains a low-strength glycolic acid.
Tone	Gently wipe your face with a hydrating toner or mist with facial water.
Eyes	Gently dot a small amount of cream around the eyes. Choose products with ingredients that address your areas of concern. Vitamin K, caffeine, vitamin C, yarrow, horse chestnut, and gingko biloba address dark circles. Haloxyl, caffeine, vitamin C, cucumber extract, green tea, and aloe vera address puffiness. Hyaluronic acid, silica, soy proteins, acai berry, aloe vera, seaweed extracts, GABA, and argireline address wrinkles, firmness, and elasticity.
Moisturize	Every evening:
	Apply a small amount of moisturizing lotion with antioxidants and vitamins.
	If you have additional skin care needs:
	Choose an oil-free moisturizer with ingredients designed to treat your specific skin care issues. Glycolic acid, tea tree oil, and zinc address oil production and breakouts. Hyaluronic acid, ceramide, olive oil, evening primrose oil, borage seed oil, colloidal oatmeal, apricot kernel oil, macadamia nut oil, safflower oil, and jojoba oil address hydration. Mulberry extract, vitamin C, pine bark extract, strawberry begonia, and magnesium ascorbyl phosphate address discoloration. Aloe vera, green tea, calendula, cucumber, chamomile, willow herb, perilla leaf extract, feverfew, evening primrose oil, red clove, mirabilis, colloidal oatmeal, red algae, and zinc address irritation and inflammation. Azelaic acid, tea tree oil, and zinc address acne flares.

INGREDIENTS TO AVOID

If your skin is excessively oily: Mineral oil, petrolatum, coconut oil

If your skin is highly sensitive: Lactic acid, glycolic acid, alpha-lipoic acid, acetic acid, benzoic acid, cinnamic acid, menthol, parabens, quaternium-15, vitamin C

If you have existing discoloration: Celery extract, lime extract, parsley extract, fig extract, carrot extract, bergamot oil, estradiol, genistein

If your skin is acne-prone: Butyl stearate, cinnamon oil, isostearyl isostearate, cocoa butter, jojoba oil, coconut oil, decyl oleate, myristyl myristate, myristyl propionate, octyl palminate, octyl stearate, peppermint oil, isopropyl stearate, isopropyl isostearate, myristate, palmitate

AT-HOME TREATMENTS

You can purchase over-the-counter masks and exfoliates for combination skin, or you can make your own (see chapter 11).

Masks	Your skin will benefit from using a mask once or twice a week to deliver hydration and high concentrations of nutrients.
Exfoliation	Using a finely textured scrub, you may exfoliate once a week to remove the top layer of dead skin cells. Don't exfoliate if you have very sensitive skin or if your acne medication causes irritation.

IN-OFFICE PROCEDURES

Cleansing facial	Hydrating facial	Microdermabrasion

DRY SKIN

MORNING REGIMEN

Step	Directions
Cleanse	Wash with a gentle, soothing, nonfoaming cleanser that contains calendula, oatmeal, or chamomile.
Tone	Mist your face with facial water that contains hyaluronic acid.
Eyes	Gently dot a small amount of cream around the eyes. Choose products with ingredients that address your areas of concern. Vitamin K, caffeine, vitamin C, yarrow, horse chestnut, and gingko biloba address dark circles. Haloxyl, caffeine, vitamin C, cucumber extract, green tea, and aloe vera address puffiness. Hyaluronic acid, silica, soy proteins, acai berry, aloe vera, seaweed extracts, GABA, and argireline address wrinkles, firmness, and elasticity.
Moisturize	Every day: 　　While your skin is still damp, apply a moisturizer that contains antioxidants. If you have additional skin care needs: 　　Choose a moisturizer with ingredients designed to treat your specific skin care issues. Ceramides, borage seed oil, canola oil, apricot kernel oil, cocoa butter (don't use if you

have acne), olive oil, glycerin, evening primrose oil, jojoba oil, macadamia nut oil, shea butter, safflower oil, colloidal oatmeal, and pumpkin seed oil address extra hydration and the ability to lock in moisture. Green tea, calendula, cucumber, aloe vera, chamomile, colloidal oatmeal, and aloe vera address irritation and inflammation. Arbutin, bearberry, coconut palm, cucumber extract, willow herb, gallic acid, hydroquinone, vitamin C, and mulberry extract address discoloration.

Protect	Apply broad-spectrum sunblock *every day*. *Note:* If your moisturizer contains a sunscreen of at least SPF 25 that blocks UVA and UVB rays, you don't need to add extra sunblock.

EVENING REGIMEN

Step	Directions
Cleanse	Wash your face with a soap-free cleanser that contains calendula, chamomile, or other soothing ingredients.
Tone	Mist your face with facial rosewater or a hydrating toner.
Eyes	Gently dot a small amount of cream around the eyes. Choose products with ingredients that address your areas of concern. Vitamin K, caffeine, vitamin C, yarrow, horse chestnut, and gingko biloba address dark circles. Haloxyl, caffeine, vitamin C, cucumber extract, green tea, and aloe vera address puffiness. Hyaluronic acid, silica, soy proteins, acai berry, aloe vera, seaweed extracts, GABA, and argireline address wrinkles, firmness, and elasticity.

Moisturize	Every evening:
	    While your skin is still damp, apply a moisturizer that contains moisture-locking ingredients like ceramides and peptides.
	
	If you have additional skin care needs:
	    Choose a moisturizer with ingredients designed to treat your specific skin care issues. Ceramides, borage seed oil, canola oil, apricot kernel oil, cocoa butter (don't use if you have acne), olive oil, glycerin, evening primrose oil, jojoba oil, macadamia nut oil, shea butter, safflower oil, colloidal oatmeal, and pumpkin seed oil address extra hydration and the ability to lock in moisture. Green tea, calendula, cucumber, aloe vera, chamomile, colloidal oatmeal, and aloe vera address irritation and inflammation. Arbutin, bearberry, coconut palm, cucumber extract, willow herb, gallic acid, hydroquinone, vitamin C, and mulberry extract address discoloration.

INGREDIENTS TO AVOID

If your skin is highly sensitive: Alcohol, lactic acid, glycolic acid, alpha-lipoic acid, acetic acid, benzoyl acid, cinnamic acid, polyhydroxy acid, phytic acid, vitamin C

If you have existing discoloration: Estradiol, estrogen, genistein, dandelion, geranium, jasmine, lavender, lemongrass, lemon oil, neroli, rose oil, tea tree oil, sandalwood

If your skin is acne-prone: Cinnamon oil, isotearyl isostearate, cocoa butter, coconut oil, peppermint oil, isopropyl myristate, isopropyl isostearate

AT-HOME TREATMENTS

You can purchase over-the-counter masks and exfoliates for dry skin, or you can make your own (see chapter 11).

Masks	Masks can hydrate, reduce irritation, and be very soothing. You can use a simple home-made mask or purchase one over the counter. When purchasing a mask, make sure it is specifically made for sensitive skin and doesn't have any of the chemicals or ingredients listed above. If you have an acne or rosacea flare, talk to your doctor before using a mask on your face or your body.
Exfoliation	Use only very gentle facial exfoliates. Avoid products with fragrances or other chemicals. Homemade scrubs are a good option. If your skin is very sensitive, you can exfoliate with dry oatmeal (see the recipe in chapter 11). Do not use any peels or microdermabrasion kits.

IN-OFFICE PROCEDURES

Cleansing facial   Hydrating facial

Menopause

BEAUTIFUL SKIN AT ANY AGE

An Emmy-winning TV actress walked into my office one day, complaining that she was having trouble getting the parts she wanted. "I know I can't play the ingenue anymore, but sometimes they won't even consider me for the part of the mom," she said. "It's not like I'm that old. After all, I'm only—" She clamped her hand over her mouth, as if she were about to reveal the code to a nuclear bomb.

Although she was probably still young enough to play (almost) any part she wanted, her skin was starting to tell a different story. As with so many women, midlife hormonal changes had left her skin looking dry and dull, aging her prematurely.

My actress patient was going through menopause, part of the life journey of every woman. The journey can be frightening if you don't know what to expect: "Am I going to grow hair all over my body?" "Am I going to turn old and wrinkly like a prune overnight?" "What's going to happen to my sex life?" More of us are going through menopause than ever before, but we have much less information about this passage than we do about the other passages in a woman's life—puberty and pregnancy. The myth is that menopause is a negative experience. The truth is, you can go through menopause and still remain feminine, attractive, sensual, and sexy.

According to gynecologist Dr. Dianne Rosenberg, at least a third of our lives takes place after the cessation of our periods. That's a lot of time to live—and to want to look *great*, and not just "great for your age." More than any other organ in our bodies, our skin is critically affected by the hormonal shifts that occur before, during, and after menopause.

My patients come to me because they need help understanding the changes that occur in their skin as the result of the hormonal process associated with menopause, and they want to know what they can do to address and minimize these changes. In this chapter you will learn:

- How menopause affects your skin
- How to heal your skin: The Dr. Ava Plan
- Strategies for minimizing the effects of menopause on your skin
- Skin-treatment options available from your health care professional
- Menopausal treatment options
- Nutrition and fitness tips for better-looking skin
- Skin care regimens for menopausal skin

The Impact of Menopause on Skin

Have you ever met someone who is young but who has really old-looking skin? Or what about the opposite: an apple-faced grandmother or even great-grandmother with the skin of someone half her years? Our skin's "age" isn't determined just by how old we are. According to a report on skin aging, a number of factors determine how well our skin ages. These include the following:

- Genetics
- History of sun exposure
- Illnesses

- Diet
- Lifestyle (work, stress)
- Alcohol and drug use
- Smoking

The report listed one other skin-aging factor: "dysfunction or aging of hormone systems"—in other words, menopause. With the loss of estrogen that occurs during menopause comes the reduced production of collagen, and this is one of the main culprits in the pathogenesis of skin aging. Collagen type 1 is responsible for skin's strength, and elastin is responsible for the skin's elastic, or resilience, properties. Some 30 percent of skin collagen is lost in the first five years after menopause, with an average decline of 2.1 percent every year thereafter. In addition, the reduced production of sebum leads to drier skin. As a result, menopause affects our skin in a number of different ways.

Acne and rosacea flares   Ironically, even as declining estrogen levels are drying your skin, the perimenopausal years—the years immediately before menopause—are like puberty in the sense that they may be marked by sharp spikes of androgen activity that trigger adult acne or rosacea flares. Midlife breakouts can be stubborn due to these hormal shifts. In addition, many acne remedies are drying or irritating to skin that is already drying out from estrogen loss. Rosacea, which is linked to inflammation, can be worsened by the vasomotor instability that causes hot flashes (more on these later).

What to do: Your first option is to try an over-the-counter remedy such as benzol peroxide, glycolic acid, salicylic acid, or perhaps even a retinol. As all of these products are drying, and your skin is most likely already dry (even though it is breaking out), always apply a moisturizer that is appropriate for your skin type. Your second option is prescription acne topical medications. These are discussed at length in chapter 8. A third option is an oral medication that blocks androgen receptors such as spironolactone, a low-dose birth control pill, or hormone-replacement therapy.

Dryness   Many women may experience skin dryness for the first time at menopause. It is one of the most common dermatological conditions affecting menopausal women. A recent study of more than thirty-eight hundred women over forty found that 36.2 percent had dry skin. Even if your skin type is naturally oily, you'll begin to notice an increased tendency toward dryness.

Skin dryness is due to three factors. There is decreased sebum (the natural skin lubricant) production, as well as an average 30 percent reduction in the natural oils of the skin. As your estrogen level drops, your skin also loses its ability to retain moisture because there are less glycosaminoglycans (GAGs) generated and the water content of the dermis is diminished. Finally, there is a defect in the water-holding capacity of the most superficial layer of the epidermis, the stratum corneum.

Studies have shown that some menopausal women may experience dryness for the first time for a very simple reason: their soap. In the same way that we change our wardrobe as we mature, we must also adjust our skin care products. A recent study showed that menopausal women had been using the same soap for decades. What may have been mild enough to use on our skin when we were younger can be very drying as we age. It may be time to change.

What to do: Switch to a nondetergent soap or use a body cleanser that has a moisturizer in it. If you are using bar soap, use it only in strategic areas (under the arms, groin, hands, and feet). Limit your time in the shower and use warm (not hot) water. After you take a shower or a bath, apply moisturizer immediately to damp skin. Look for a moisturizer that is more occlusive or feels slightly greasy. Another tip is to mix a couple of spoonfuls of oil in with your moisturizer (sesame, coconut, jojoba, olive). Wait five minutes before dressing to give it a chance to soak in. If your skin is dry and cracking, there are prescription moisturizers available from your health care provider (brand names: *Epiceram*, *Tetrix*, *Eletone*).

Dullness   Fluctuating hormone levels during perimenopause promote the buildup of sticky dead skin cells in your pores. Later, as hormone levels decline, your skin's natural turnover cycle slows down. Dry skin flakes aren't sloughed off as readily, which leads to a dull, sometimes ashen appearance.

What to do: Since the dullness is due to an uneven surface, the use of at-home exfoliation, masks, scrubs, and peels in your skin care program will bring the light back to your face.

Eye irritation   Your eyelids also have oil-producing glands whose function is to provide oil to the tear film to keep it from evaporating. Estrogen loss affects these oil glands, too, and your eyes may become dry, irritated, and red. It's important to attend to your dry eyes in the same way you attend to the rest of your body, as severe dry eye can damage your cornea and lead to vision loss.

What to do: Start with over-the-counter artificial tears and put them in frequently. If you don't get any relief, a prescription medication may help.

> **DR. AVA'S MYTH BREAKER**
>
> **The myth:** Women look for solutions to the aging effects of menopause because they are vain, in a futile hunt for lost youth, or just to please a man.
>
> **The truth:** These attitudes reflect a bias against women choosing to be healthy and beautiful at any age. In my experience, women at midlife want to look beautiful and feel sexually confident. They're intent on celebrating the mature present and living into a healthy future. They seek help from me to look fantastic at all times.

Fat redistribution   The changing contours of your face at midlife aren't just a product of collagen and elastin loss or wrinkling. As your estrogen level drops (and the long-term effects of gravity kick in), the fat pads that gave your face a youthful roundness begin to thin out and move down, creating hollows under your eyes or sagging jowls along your jawline.

What to do: Visit a health care practitioner who is proficient in the use of injectables to revolumize the face (brand names: *Juvederm, Restylane, Sculptra, Perlane, Radiesse*).

Fine lines, wrinkles, and textural changes   Estrogen loss contributes to the development of fine surface lines as well as deeper lines caused by motion (for example, frown and smile lines and crow's feet). The skin on your cheeks may develop a rippled appearance, like crepe paper.

What to do: Look for skin care products that contain alpha-hydroxy acids, retinol, antioxidants, and peptides. AHA will gently exfoliate the skin, giving it a polished appearance. Retinols will also exfoliate the skin and at the same time stimulate collagen production, which is a gradual process, so don't expect overnight results. Because your skin's reservoir of its own antioxidants is depleted in menopause, their replacement can help firm the skin by preventing further oxidative damage from environmental exposure. Peptides can help relax the muscles responsible for lines caused by motion, and some stimulate collagen production. If the lines are still bothersome, visit your health care professional for a consultation regarding the use of neuromodulators or fillers to correct the deeper lines.

Hair   Changes in hair color and texture often herald the beginning of your perimenopause. Your hair texture may change, and your hair may thin (not only on your scalp but also on other parts of your body). In addition, fluctuating levels of androgen during perimenopause may convert some of the fine hairs on your face to wirier, darker hairs, particularly above your upper lip and on your chin.

What to do: See your doctor for a full evaluation. Hair thinning can be caused by thyroid disease, anemia, and connective tissue disease. Hair loss due to hormonal changes is a diagnosis after all other conditions are ruled out. Treatment options include topical minoxidil, oral supplements such as biotin, and on occasion an oral androgen blocker such as spironolactone.

Hot flashes and night sweats   The symptoms of a thousand lame jokes, these are probably the conditions we most associate with menopause. It is the episodic, unpredictable, recurrent day or night precipitous sweating that is said to occur in more than half of all perimenopausal and menopausal women in the United States.

Sweating is the result of hormone-triggered changes in the body's internal thermostat. You're most likely to experience hot flashes during the last part of perimenopause, when your brain is kicking out higher and higher levels of the hormones associated with ovulation in a vain attempt to get the ovaries to respond.

Even though the chief cause is an internal vasomotor (circulation) imbalance, hot flashes can be triggered or made worse by outside factors such as stress, heat, spicy foods, and alcohol.

"This is a bit of a catch-22," explains Dr. Rosenberg. "Many women like to have a glass of wine to help them relax. However, since drinking alcohol causes vasodilation, flushing can occur. Having a glass of wine can actually exacerbate hot flashes, which wind up making the perimenopausal/menopausal woman feel worse."

There also seems to be a connection between hot flashes and menopausal rosacea flares.

What to do: There are many different herbal remedies that help some people with hot flashes. Certainly hormone replacement therapy will eliminate this menopausal problem. Discuss with your doctor what option is best for you.

Itching   Dry, flaky skin—a result of estrogen depletion—can itch. If you scratch the itch, you may trigger more itching and irritation. In fact, some women become more likely to develop contact dermatitis or hives after menopause, when hormone-related changes to the immune system trigger hypersensitivity.

If you think your perimenopausal symptoms are driving you buggy, you're not wrong. Many women experience a nerve-related sensation that is best described as having bugs crawling under the skin, often in conjunction with hot flashes.

What to do: Address all of your dry skin issues with moisturizers, as discussed earlier. If your skin is still itchy, try an over-the-counter nondrowsy antihistamine such as Claritin or Zyrtec or visit your health care professional.

Lips   Your lips are replete with oil-producing glands whose output is similarly diminished by estrogen depletion. Over the years cumulative sun exposure can damage the lip epidermis, contributing to dryness that can cause peeling. In fact, if you have participated in an outdoor sport such as tennis, skiing, or running and have constantly peeling lips, you may have *actinic cheilitis*, a precancerous condition that needs to be treated by your doctor.

What to do: Use a lip balm that has ceramides and SPF and is fragrance-free to both treat and protect the area. Wear lipstick! It can help moisturize the lips depending on the formulation. If peeling persists, see your physician to make sure that neither sun damage nor an allergic reaction is the cause.

Nails   As the rest of your skin gets drier with hormone depletion, so do your nails. You may notice vertical ridges on your nails, and the nails may become more fragile and susceptible to peeling, splitting, or breaking. Cuticles dry out more easily, too, leading to torn cuticles and hangnails.

What to do: Limit your exposure to water by wearing protective gloves for housework. In the evening, try massaging almond oil into your nails and cuticles. Apply an AHA-containing moisturizer and wear a pair of cotton gloves to bed. If you wear nail polish, use the less drying non-acetone nail polish remover. Some people have found a biotin supplement to be helpful.

Pigmentation changes   Fluctuating levels of estrogen and progesterone during perimenopause can trigger the pigment-producing cells in your skin to shift into overdrive, causing skin to pigment unevenly. You might develop melasma, a darkening of the skin across your cheekbones, upper lip, and forehead that is also common (for the same hormonal reasons) during pregnancy. As your estrogen level drops, your skin becomes more sensitive to UV radiation, darkening existing brown spots or developing new ones. Sun damage and chronological aging are also at work in the development of the flat tan lesions known as *age spots* or *liver spots*.

What to do: Begin with prevention. Wear sunscreen every day regardless of rain or sun, whether you are indoors or outdoors. Keep a hat in your purse, not sitting in your closet. At-home treatments to even out your skin tone include skin lighteners such as hydroquinone, arbutin, and kojic acid. Retinols and glycolic acid also improve melasma because they exfoliate the skin and even out the pigment layer (brand names: *Triluna, Glytone*). In general, physical exfoliation should be avoided because the paradoxical result of further skin darkening can occur. In-office procedures are limited to peels because lasers or intense pulsed light devices tend to worsen the situation.

Sagging   Midlife hormonal changes affect the production of collagen and the elastin fibers that together give skin its tensile strength, elasticity, and underlying support. The skin thus becomes thinner, and when combined with underlying skeletal changes, loss of supportive facial fat pads leads to sagging. You may first notice this effect on your eyelids, where skin is thinnest and has the least underlying support.

What to do: Replacing volume requires an in-office procedure so that the skin can drape over the restored volume in a more youthful fashion, using injectables such as Restylane, Juvaderm, or Radiesse. However, keep in mind that when your skin is in the best condition possible, you will still look good.

Thinness and transparency Your skin thickens little by little each year until you reach your forties. Then the process reverses because of decreases in collagen, water, and GAGs. Because your skin becomes thinner and more fragile, you may notice more frequent cuts, bruises, and transparency. These phenomena may occur more on your arms, chest, and neck than your face.

What to do: The ideal choice is a serum containing vitamin C along with a retinol or a prescription Retin-A. A compounding pharmacy can also add vitamin K, which in some people can help with bruising. As the skin on the neck and chest tends to be more delicate, reduce possible irritation from active ingredients by mixing serum and moisturizer together before applying or by applying moisturizer immediately on top of serum. Know that it takes time to see improvement.

> **DR. AVA'S SKINFORMATION**
>
> Although the thinning of skin that accompanies estrogen loss makes wound healing slower, there's an upside. Thin skin is less likely to develop excessive scarring, so when wounds do heal, they'll leave fewer marks behind. Also, if you had a tendency to develop keloids (fibrous tissue) in your younger years, you may find that menopause greatly reduces their formation.

Healing Your Skin: The Dr. Ava Plan

At this point in your busy life, your skin is multitasking and so are you. Maybe you're running a successful business, or maybe you've decided to go back to school. Maybe you're still taking care of your adult children and now you're also looking after your aging parents. You've got responsibility for pets and a home, and you're running a support group for everyone in your life.

With that in mind, you need your skin care plan to be simple and effective. For example, exfoliation sloughs off the dry skin cells that accumulate as a result of hormonal changes, but you don't have to do it every day. It's not written in stone that you have to do it only in the morning or only at night. You have to figure out what products work best for your skin type and when it's best to use them. Now is the time to make taking care of your skin a top priority. Once you get into a routine, you'll find that it's surprisingly easy to do.

As we've already discussed, the effects of estrogen depletion on women's skin are multiple. These changes include thinning of the epidermis (the top layer of the skin), decrease in the collagen content, diminished moisture, and decreased elasticity. Wound healing has been shown to take a longer amount of time.

The underlying cause of these changes is multifactorial. One factor is the direct effect of lower estrogen levels. Another is the senescence, or aging, of the fibroblasts, the skin cells that reside in the dermis. These are the manufacturing centers for the proteins collagen, which gives skin its firmness, and elastin, which gives it the snap-back quality. When the cells get old, they make less elastin and collagen. The lower amounts of these structural proteins give skin its thin, flaccid appearance instead of the plumpness and firmness associated with youth and premenopausal hormone levels.

In other words, your skin is on a hormonal roller coaster. It's essential that you follow a skin care program that gives your skin support and stimulation as it rides the twists and turns of that roller coaster.

Phase 1: Cleanse and Exfoliate

To cleanse your skin, keep in mind one simple rule: you're already dry, so don't overdo it. However, in order for active nutrients to penetrate to the level of skin where they are needed (the dermis), you will still have to gently remove dead cells from the top layer of your skin. That means addressing both issues as you clean your skin morning and night.

Because your skin is dry, use only cleansers designed for dry or sensitive skin. Make sure they are not loaded with fragrances or coloring, because they can be damaging or irritating. Never pick one that foams;

it may contain detergents or other harsh chemicals. If you like, you can use two different cleansers: one in the morning that hydrates and one in the evening that soothes. If your skin is slightly oily or if you have break-outs, choose a cleanser with an AHA or salicylic acid, because these provide an additional level of gentle exfoliation.

In addition to the dryness caused by estrogen depletion, midlife skin can look dull because the turnover of dead skin cells slows down with age. Dry skin looks leathery and doesn't reflect light, which makes you look older. If your skin isn't overly sensitive or inflamed with acne or rosacea, exfoliate every day to clear the dulling surface layer of dead cells. Exfoliation also improves circulation, allows better penetration of nutrients and hydration into your skin's deeper layers, and reduces the appearance of fine lines and the dark spots of sun damage.

To exfoliate, you can:

- Cleanse your face and then wipe it firmly with a damp terry cloth washcloth. The roughened surface will remove some dead skin cells.
- Or, use a facial nylon puff or a disposable nylon pad moistened with cleanser. Wipe your face with a gentle but firm circular motion. Avoid the very thin skin around your eyes. For the body, use a soft loofah (a natural sea sponge) or a large nylon puff in the bath or shower.
- Use a home exfoliation and/or microdermabrasion device. These range from battery-operated pore cleansers gentle enough for use on acne-prone skin (brand names: *Dove, Zia, Pretika)* to sonic brushes for deep cleansing (brand names: *Clarisonic, Pretika*). You can usually find a variety of disposable pads and sponges or inter-changeable brush heads to suit your skin type.

You may also want to choose skin care products that include exfoli-ating ingredients. Cleansers and masks that contain exfoliants are often called scrubs (brand names: *Neutrogena Body Clear Body Scrub, 100% Pure Organic Fuji Apple Body Scrub, Cellex-C Speed Peel Body Polish*).

The most common exfoliating ingredients are:

- **Physical exfoliants** Salt crystals, oatmeal, crushed nut shells or apricot kernels, pumice, or tiny plastic beads can be used as home exfoliants. These ingredients can also be found in many commercially prepared masks and scrubs. I don't recommend the plastic beads, also known as "mermaid's tears," because they don't biodegrade and can harm marine life.

- **Alpha-hydroxy acid**   AHAs such as glycolic acid, lactic acid, and malic acid are among the most effective exfoliating ingredients. Because AHAs are water-soluble, they can penetrate deeper into the skin's surface to lift off dead cells. They have some moisturizing properties, too, but they may irritate sensitive skin if they are used in too high a concentration.
- **Polyhydroxy acids**   PHAs are a new generation of AHAs, designed to be gentle and penetrate the skin more slowly. This makes them better suited for use by people with sensitive skin. PHAs include lactobionic acid, galactose, and gluconic acid.
- **Salicylic acid**   Salicylic acid, obtained from willow bark, is a beta-hydroxy acid. It also serves as an exfoliant and is particularly effective at breaking up the sticky gum of dead cells and sebum that blocks pores and causes acne flares. Because salicylic acid is fat-soluble, it doesn't penetrate below the epidermis.

Phase 2: Nourish

Your body needs nutrients to stay healthy and strong, and so does your skin, especially now that midlife hormonal changes have presented you with some new and interesting skin-related challenges. One of the biggest challenges is the ongoing battle against free radicals (see chapter 3), which cause damage to collagen, elastin, and other delicate skin components. The damage is exacerbated by the loss of hormonal protection at midlife.

The most effective way to fight free radicals is by adding antioxidants to your diet and skin care program. Antioxidants are vitamins and minerals that basically disarm free radicals, giving your skin an opportunity to fight the existing damage (such as redness and brown spots) and return to its healthy glow. When choosing skin care products, look for these antioxidants:

- **Vitamin C**   The ascorbic acid found in citrus fruits and leafy vegetables helps prevent the aging effect of UV damage and is required for collagen formation.
- **Green tea polyphenols**   These antioxidants fight inflammation.
- **Vitamin E**   Alpha-tocopherol, sometimes combined with ferulic acid, assists with wound healing and prevents melanin formation.
- **Alpha-lipoic acid**   Along with its variant, dihydrolipoic acid (DHLA), this improves the signs of aging.
- **Coffeeberry**   An extract of the coffee plant *C. arabica*, this is an anti-inflammatory that reduces skin irritation and pigment changes and has a rejuvenating effect.
- **Pomegranate extract**   This helps prevent photoaging, is a strong antioxidant, and can even out pigmentation.
- **Grape seed extract**   This fights inflammation and can increase skin moisture content.
- **Coenzyme Q10**   Also known as ubiquinone, this supports the formation of collagen and elastin.
- **Pycnogenol**   A standardized extract of pine bark, this improves skin elasticity and texture.
- **Silymarin**   A flavonoid compound obtained from milk thistle seeds, this has anti-inflammatory properties and prevents UV damage.
- **Niacinamide**   Niacinamide (also known as nicotinamide), a derivative of vitamin B_3, improves photodamage and is used to treat roscea.
- **Resveratrol**   A compound found in grape skins and seeds, berries, peanuts, and red wine, this ingredient may extend cell life.
- **Genistein**   A soy isoflavone, this helps even out the pigment layer.

> **DR. AVA'S SKINFORMATION**
>
> If you add some of the following antioxidant-rich foods to your diet, your skin will thank you: applesauce, artichoke, asparagus, avocado, beets, bell peppers, black-eyed peas, blueberries, broccoli, brussels sprouts, cherries, chili powder, cilantro, cinnamon, cloves, cocoa, cranberries, dates, eggplant, fuji apples, ginger, green tea, kale, nuts, oatmeal, oranges, papaya, parsley, peaches, pears, plums, red cabbage, spinach, and tangerines. For a more complete list, see chapter 5.

Phase 3: Moisturize

As estrogen depletion begins to take its drying toll on your skin, it's important to fight back with an effective moisturizing routine. Your routine will help your skin on two levels: adding moisture to dry skin cells and preventing the loss of internal moisture.

Keep in mind that if you're experiencing adult acne flares during perimenopause, your moisturizing needs will be different from someone who is experiencing age-related dryness and fine wrinkling. It is important to choose ingredients and formulations geared to your age, skin type, and specific skin issues (brand names: *Aveeno, CeraVe, Vanicream, Avene, Skinceuticals, Eucerin, Jergens, Vanilla, La Roche-Posay Lipid Replenishing Body Milk*). See the skin care regimens at the end of this chapter for other recommendations).

There is always a dizzying array of moisturizing options at any skin care counter. However, look for these proven moisturizing ingredients:

- **Humectants**   These include glycerin, urea, lactic acid, and hyaluronic acid. Humectants attract moisture from the environment as well as the dermis, increasing water content in the skin and temporarily reducing the appearance of fine lines.
- **Occlusives**   These include lanolin, oils, petrolatum, and silicone derivatives. Occlusives block moisture evaporation by forming a film on the skin's surface, helping to make the skin appear smoother by locking in moisture.
- **Emollients**   These include ceramides, fatty acids, and lipids such as shea butter and oatmeal. Emollients fill in the cracks between the skin cells, sealing them together to improve skin texture and the skin's barrier function.

Phase 4: Rejuvenate

One of the most visible signs of estrogen depletion is the loss of skin firmness that results from the slowdown in collagen and elastin production. You can't entirely reverse this process, but there are skin care ingredients that have been shown to stimulate cell growth and promote collagen repair. The following list includes proven anti-aging ingredients in skin care products.

Retinol   A derivative of vitamin A, this has been proven to promote skin cell turnover and collagen production, repair elastin, and reverse other effects of photoaging. Retinol's effects are dosage-related. Over-the-counter formulations may contain very low dosages that don't have significant effects. Prescription treatments may contain dosages high enough to be irritating to sensitive skin—but they will cause skin cell turnover. All retinoids have the potential to cause dryness, redness, and peeling, especially in the first few days of use.

Peptides   These are short chains of amino acids that can have various effects on skin cells. The best anti-aging peptides have been shown to stimulate collagen production, reduce collagen destruction, thicken the epidermis (reducing skin thinning and leading to better wound healing), and even out pigmentation. As with retinol, the effects of peptides depend on the amount. If the peptide is listed in the bottom third of ingredients on a product label, the product doesn't contain enough to make a difference.

Collagen and peptides   Both are often included in moisturizers for their supposed anti-aging qualities. Neither true humectants nor occlusives, they leave a thin film on the surface of the skin that provides a temporary tightening and smoothing effect and seals in some moisture.

Natural ingredients   Oatmeal and shea butter may be included in skin care products because they have proven moisturizing benefits. Oatmeal contains lipids that prevent transepidermal water loss (TEWL). It has the ability to hydrate skin by binding to water. Shea butter is an

---

DR. AVA'S MYTH BREAKER

The myth: Using creams or lotions that contain collagen will reduce wrinkles and replenish your skin's collagen.

The truth: Although there are active ingredients that you can apply topically to stimulate collagen production, collagen, ironically, isn't one of them. Collagen molecules are generally too large to penetrate deep into the dermis, and even when they're micronized, there's no proof that they are incorporated into the skin's own collagen production cycle. Don't toss your topical collagen formulas, however, because the collagen molecules in them do serve to lock in moisture.

emollient produced from the nut of an African tree. It is high in moisturizing fats and also has some anti–inflammatory properties.

For information on professional rejuvenation treatments, see the section on treating menopausal skin at the doctor's office.

Phase 5: Protect

I tell my patients that no matter where they are in the menopause process—just starting, in the middle, or enjoying their postmenopausal years—there is one major step that's never too late to take to drastically improve the appearance of their skin: protect it from the sun. Skin that's been protected from UV damage will be far less likely to show the aging effects of hormonal depletion. Although your skin will be drier after menopause, it won't be leathery. You'll have fine lines but few deep wrinkles. Your skin tone will be more even, with fewer dark patches, age spots, or other pigmentation problems.

Apply a sunscreen or sunblock with an SPF of at least 25 and combined UVA and UVB protection every day, no matter what the weather. Make sure your UV protection is appropriate for your skin type and won't cause your skin to break out or clog your pores.

For dry skin, try Neutrogena Sensitive Sunblock, Aveeno Continuous Protection, or Eucerin Sensitive Facial Skin Lotion. Neutrogena and Eucerin also make a sunblock for oily skin, and Aveeno makes a product for combination skin. Lips also need UV protection (brand names: *DDF Glossy Lip Therapy, Fallene LIPCoTZ, Bioelements Instant Lip Emollient, Avene Lip Balm, Dr. Haruschka Lip Care Stick*).

ASK DR. AVA

I've been really good about sunscreen and all that, but I look so pale and I want to get some color. Is it okay to use a tanning booth?

In a word, no. You're still damaging your skin whether you're tanning on the beach or in a booth. Today there are great self-tanning options in the form of tinted moisturizers or self-tanning creams. No more excuses for baking yourself.

While you're slathering on the sunscreen, don't forget to cover up with clothing, especially wide-brimmed hats and long-sleeved shirts. Wear sunglasses; large, wraparound styles with green-tinted lenses that block UV rays provide the best protection. Be sure to check your vitamin D levels with a blood test at your health care provider's office. If your levels are low, you may need to take a supplement.

Healing Menopausal Skin

Along with the Dr. Ava Skin Care Plan, there are other strategies you can follow to dramatically improve your skin during the menopausal years. Some of these can be done at home, but others will require a visit to the doctor's office.

At Home

The most important thing you can do at home is to examine how your lifestyle (and any bad habits) might be affecting the health of your skin—and what you can do to change it. Here are some suggestions:

Get rid of the cigarettes. Do you really need to hear this from me? Quit now, if not for your health, then for your vanity. Smoking is almost as damaging to your skin as UV radiation is.

Get your weight under control. As you move into menopause, your metabolism will slow down, making it harder to burn off calories. The shift in fat distribution that accompanies estrogen withdrawal can put excess strain on your internal organs and your peripheral circulation, which can also increase the possibility of varicose veins. There are drawbacks to being underweight as well, of course, or to dieting excessively during and after menopause. If you are too thin, you may look older than you really are or be at risk for osteoporosis. Work with your health care professional or dietitian now to develop a healthy eating plan that will take you through menopause.

Get fit. Regular exercise is probably more important now than at any other time in your life. Not only does it help you to keep your weight within a healthy range, it also alleviates many perimenopausal symptoms.

Get help managing chronic diseases and other medical or dental conditions. If you're living with diabetes, rheumatoid arthritis, or any other ongoing health challenge, it's important to be rigorous in complying with your treatment plan. That goes for dental health and hygiene, too.

Get into a routine. If you've been practicing good skin care all your life, it won't be difficult to make the necessary adjustments to compensate for the effects of menopause. If you haven't done much more than run a comb through your hair and add a dab of lipstick, now is the time to learn how to care for your skin; it's easy.

At the Doctor's Office

Your doctor can offer a variety of additional noninvasive treatment options for refreshing and rejuvenating hormonally challenged skin. These include:

Topicals   Your doctor may prescribe a variety of different topical treatments, depending on which skin-related menopausal symptom you are trying to address:

- **Dry skin**   Brand names: *Epiceram Cream, Eletone, Mimyx*
- **Brown spots or sun damage**   Brand names: *Renova, Tazorac, Tretinoin, TriLuma*
- **Rosacea**   Brand names: *Finacea, Metrogel*
- **Acne breakouts**   Brand names: *Epiduo, Ziana, Triaz, Atralin*

Peels   Peels are a form of accelerated exfoliation that use a chemical to remove one or more layers of the skin's surface, exposing new skin cells and promoting a more rapid turnover of dead cells. Peels reduce the appearance of fine lines and make skin look brighter and younger.

The chemicals used in peels include glycolic acid, trichloroacetic acid, salicylic acid, lactic acid, and carbolic acid (phenol). Depending on the concentration, the peel may be light, medium, or deep in intensity. Deep peels provide the most visible results but also involve more downtime because of redness and swelling. Your doctor or aesthetician will advise you how to prepare your skin for a chemical peel and what follow-up steps to take. With even the lightest peels, as with any exfoliation, you will need to avoid UV exposure while the new skin is still particularly vulnerable.

Laser treatments   Originally used to correct birthmarks and pigmentation problems and to reduce acne scarring, lasers have become popular weapons in the anti-aging battle. In my practice I've pioneered many of these laser procedures, which have now become standard in cosmetic dermatology. Laser peels use the controlled application of heat to resurface the skin, either superficially or at the deeper dermal levels. There are three broad categories of lasers:

- **Ablative resurfacing lasers**   These are used to reduce deep wrinkles and hyperpigmentation, stimulate collagen growth, and speed cell regeneration. They remove the top layer of the skin. This treatment requires significant downtime. Ablative lasers include the Erbium:YAG and carbon dioxide (CO_2).

- **Fractionated lasers**   These are used to improve texture, fine lines and wrinkles, and acne scars and may stimulate some tissue tightening. Depending on whether they are *ablative* or *nonablative*, you may experience some swelling or redness with minimal downtime or raw oozing skin that can require as long as a week for recuperation (brand names: *Fraxel, Active FX, Palomar*).

- **Nonablative lasers**   These are used to improve the appearance of age spots and fine lines without significant downtime. Nonablative lasers include Smoothbeam, intense pulsed light, and Q-switched ruby lasers for reduction of brown spots, and Cynosure and Candela Vbeam for reduction of broken blood vessels and redness. These lasers are also useful in treating midlife acne and rosacea flares.

Radio-frequency tissue tightening   Radio-frequency treatments use radio waves to superheat the skin's underlying tissues while keeping the surface cool. This immediately tightens skin and stimulates collagen production and tissue remodeling, making it useful for treating acne scarring. There are new fractionated radio-frequency devices. This procedure does not have the downtime of peels or ablative lasers (brand names: *Thermage, Accent, eMatrix*).

Neuromodulators   Under the brand names Botox Cosmetic and Dysport, botulinum toxin (BTX) has developed a well-deserved reputation as a first-line weapon in the fight against the signs of skin aging. It is particularly effective in treating the so-called dynamic wrinkles that develop in the skin over muscles of expression. When injected intramuscularly at specific sites, BTX relaxes the muscles, preventing the overlying skin from moving and thereby smoothing out wrinkled surfaces.

Neuromodulators are most commonly used to do the following:

- Treat wrinkling of the upper face, especially the forehead
- Lessen crow's feet (wrinkling at the corners of the eyes)
- Provide a temporary brow lift

BTX can also be used to soften the "marionette" lines that run from the outside corners of the mouth to the jaw, to alleviate the deep wrinkling that smokers develop around the mouth, and to relax the muscle bands in the neck that give it a "turkey" appearance.

Administered correctly—by a professional who uses a calculated dosage at a proper injection site—BTX carries very little risk of complication. The complications that can occur are transient and may include bruising at the injection site.

> ## DR. AVA'S SKIN SAVERS
>
> To lower the risk of bruising with injectables, talk to your physician about avoiding the use of aspirin, nonsteroidal anti-inflammatory drugs like ibuprofen, or any other blood-thinning medications for ten days before treatment.

Injectable dermal fillers   To treat deeper wrinkles and compensate for structural volume loss, dermatologists and plastic surgeons use a variety of injectable dermal fillers. These are substances that can be injected into and underneath the skin to fill out depressions and create a smoother, more youthful appearance. Think of fillers as scaffolding that holds up a building whose underlying structures have begun to sag a bit.

Right now there are several types of facial filler:

Hyaluronic acid   According to statistics from the American Academy of Aesthetic Plastic Surgeons, nearly one and a half million patients were treated with HA in 2007 alone. Popular injectable HA (brand names: *Restylane, Perlane, Juvederm*) is formulated in the laboratory. HA doesn't cause allergic reactions, so it does not require skin testing. Various brands and formulations of HA perform differently and are best suited to different areas of the face but can also be used in the hands. HA treatments have been shown to stimulate collagen, and the initial effect lasts from four to twelve months. A pleasing effect persists after repeated treatments.

Radiesse   Made of synthetic calcium-based microspheres suspended in water-based gels, this product is used to restore volume and for facial contouring. Radiesse provides immediate visual improvement. The substance also triggers new collagen formation.

Sculptra   Made of poly-L-lactic acid, which is a biocompatible and biodegradable synthetic material, this product is a tissue stimulator. Sculptra is effective for restoring facial fullness and does so in a gradual fashion over several months time through a series of treatments.

Autologous fat transfer   Fat has been used as a cosmetic filler solution for more than a century. In this procedure, which is also known as lipotransfer, fat cells are surgically harvested from the patient's thighs or abdomen and injected into the face to plump up the volume. After the initial injection, the remaining cells can be frozen and injected later. Because this treatment uses your own cells (that's what *autologous* means), there is no risk of allergy. Nevertheless, it is invasive, carries the risk of infection, and can be time-consuming. In some people the transfer lasts for months; for a lucky few, it lasts for years. Lipotransfer is a surgical procedure and *must* be performed *only* by an experienced physician.

Surgical options   Though beyond the scope of this book, surgical rejuvenation solutions continue to provide satisfaction for some people. However, the procedures are more costly, are invasive, may have more complications, and require longer recovery times.

Medical Treatments for Menopause

According to gynecologist Dr. Rosenberg, the most important thing your doctor can do for you during this time is to listen to you.

"Sometimes a patient will tell me her body has been inhabited by a demon," she says, "and it may feel that way. The hormone instability associated with menopause can start as early as thirty-five. A patient's hormones can ebb and surge all day long or all week long or both. Ninety percent of treating this process involves taking a patient's history. What is bothering her? Is it night sweats? Dry skin? Decreased libido? Vaginal dryness? Insomnia? Headaches? It is important to validate how the patient is

Menopausal Skin Care

A CASE STUDY

"I'm Afraid to Look in the Mirror"

Patient: Andrea, Caucasian, late forties

Andrea came to me complaining that her skin was looking "less alive," and it had an almost grayish tint to it. She told me that every morning when she woke up, she was afraid to look in the mirror because it seemed that she had developed a new line or wrinkle overnight! "There's always some new problem going on with my skin, and I just can't get it under control these days." Andrea had been divorced for a few years, but her appearance made her feel insecure about dating again.

Treatment Plan

I asked Andrea if she was in menopause yet. Yes, she was, she said, according to her ob-gyn. I explained that all of the changes going on with her skin, though frustrating, were part of that menopause process and something we could certainly address with different treatments and an updated skin care plan.

My first goal was to help Andrea improve her skin's texture, color, tone, and quality. We began with a chemical peel that had an exfoliating effect, removing the top grayish layer of skin. Next, Andrea had a radio-frequency treatment to boost collagen production and give her skin more elasticity. Finally, she had a Fraxel laser treatment to decrease some of the fine lines and wrinkles she was finding in the mirror every morning. I also adjusted her skin care plan, because she'd been using the same products since her twenties! Now it was time for her to adopt a less drying approach by switching to a gentler cleanser, hydrating serum, and moisturizer.

For additional skin rejuvenation, I prescribed Retin-A for her to use at night, and I suggested that she help her skin to fight free radicals with a fitness program and a change in her diet to one filled with fruits, vegetables, and high-quality protein and carbohydrates. I was happy to hear that she felt so good about how she looked that she felt confident enough to start dating again!

feeling, identify her unique constellation of symptoms, and be familiar with her personal and familial medical history." After that, Dr. Rosenberg adds, "You and your doctor will decide on the best treatment plan."

When a woman is coping with these new and unwelcome conditions, there are two basic treatment options: nonhormonal or hormonal. Although hormonal solutions are controversial, they do provide short-term relief for most of the problematic perimenopausal symptoms. According to Dr. Rosenberg, there are various types of hormonal treatment regimens.

Oral Contraceptives

Because so many annoying perimenopausal symptoms are caused by the fluctuation of hormone levels, some women find relief in stabilizing their hormone levels by continuing or starting the use of oral contraceptives. The birth control pill regulates the monthly cycle, thus suppressing the firestorm of conflicting hormonal signals that accompany perimenopause.

The FDA has approved use of the Pill only for contraception, but during perimenopause, the Pill can also:

- Regularize an irregular menstrual cycle
- Control excessive menstrual bleeding
- Reduce symptoms linked to hormonal fluctuation, like hot flashes, insomnia, mood swings, and memory problems
- Suppress adult acne flares
- Help prevent bone loss
- Decrease the tendency to develop fibrocystic breast tissue
- Prevent vaginal dryness
- Slow drying and wrinkling of skin

As you approach menopause, your doctor may recommend transitioning you from the birth control pill to an estrogen and progesterone regimen for your age. These regimens are referred to as *hormone replacement therapy*, or *HRT*, and have lower doses of hormones than birth control pills.

Hormone Replacement Therapy

Hormone replacement therapy in general remains controversial, and recommendations change frequently as new studies are published. You need to know what you are taking and how long to remain on treatment. "The reality is once you taper off, you may experience symptoms again," Dr. Rosenberg says. "Your symptoms, personal and family history of risk factors such as heart disease and breast cancer will determine the length of your treatment."

There are many claims made about different tests that can be given to determine the ideal formula necessary to regain your premenopausal hormonal equilibrium. Because hormonal levels fluctuate throughout the day, a blood test taken at ten in the morning doesn't necessarily reflect your hormonal status at three in the afternoon. In general, saliva tests are also unreliable. Therefore, the dose and type of HRT regimen selected for every individual patient is often a trial-and-error process based on laboratory analysis *and* symptom evaluation. This process can take a few months before arriving at an ideal dose and combination. After initiating HRT, most physicians will monitor symptoms and check blood tests to evaluate hormone levels.

If you are a candidate for HRT, there is a menu of choices to consider:

Which hormones?   HRT involves the use of estrogen, progesterone, or a combination of the two. If estrogen is prescribed, then it is usually accompanied by progesterone. Recent studies support the use of "natural progesterone" as opposed to a "synthetic progestin," because it appears to be safer and may have other health benefits. Sleepiness is a side effect of natural progesterone, and it should be taken at bedtime. For many women, this side effect helps to manage perimenopausal/menopausal-associated insomnia. The main purpose of adding progesterone to estrogen therapy is to prevent endometrial hyperplasia, an overgrowth of the uterine lining that is no longer being shed through menstruation, and is advisable if you still have a uterus. Your gynecologist may periodically monitor the lining of your uterus with ultrasound or biopsy to confirm there is no overgrowth. "If you have any abnormal bleeding after menopause, both procedures should be performed. Occasionally hysteroscopy is necessary for further evaluation," says Dr. Rosenberg.

Which delivery system?   Pills or creams? In pill form, hormones pass through the liver first, which can lead to a higher risk of systemic side effects. Topical creams, gels, transdermal patches, and estrogen supplied by vaginal rings are absorbed through the skin and don't pass first through the liver. They present fewer risks but also deliver lower dosages. Your choice will depend on the severity and type of your symptoms and your general health profile.

Bioidentical?   There's been a lot of attention paid recently to the source of the hormones in HRT. Bioidentical hormones are typically derived from plant sources like yams and soy and then processed to become structurally identical to the hormones made by the human body. This approach is no different from what is used for most commercially available postmenopausal hormone preparations (with the exception of urine-derived conjugated estrogens). Neither formulation is completely "natural" because both are synthesized in the laboratory. Bioidentical hormones may have an emotional appeal because of trends toward the concept of "natural products." Current medical literature does not support that bioidentical hormones have any advantage over conventional hormonal therapies.

Compounded?   Please be aware that bioidentical and individually compounded HRT preparations are not synonymous. An established compounding pharmacy recommended to you by your physician can provide HRT in the form of creams, gels, suppositories, or lozenges, and can be quite effective. Most physicians check their patients' hormone levels by a blood test before and after receiving HRT, in addition to monitoring their symptoms. These formulations are by prescription only, but be aware that individually compounded hormones aren't regulated by the FDA.

Dr. Wendy's Eating Well during Menopause

A plant-based diet that is rich in bright and colorful vegetables and fruits, whole grains, legumes, lean meat, and low-fat dairy contributes to a clear and glowing complexion. This diet has also been shown to reduce the risk of heart disease and diabetes, both of which pose extra risks to post-menopausal women.

As estrogen dips, a nutrient-rich diet becomes even more important to support the moisture and the integrity of the skin. It can be helpful to include foods that contain phytoestrogens—naturally occurring weak estrogen-like compounds—as part of a well-balanced diet over time. Dr. Rosenberg cautions that it can take three to six months to see the benefits from phytoestrogens in a woman's chemistry and to check with your physician.

The following foods contain phytoestrogens and are also collagen-friendly:

- Soybeans (edamame)
- Soy nuts
- Ground flaxseed
- Walnuts
- Tofu
- Tempeh
- Soy milk (low-fat, calcium-enriched, and unsweetened preferred)
- Bioflavonoid-rich foods like cherries, cranberries, blueberries, bilberries, grape skins, and many whole grains
- The soft inner peel of citrus fruits

For some women, soy—especially processed soy foods (like those found in meat substitutes and energy bars that contain soy protein isolates)—is not recommended. Check with your primary-care doctor or oncologist for specific advice.

Moisturize from the Inside Out: Drink—and Eat—Your Water

Water plays an essential role in virtually every function in the body, from keeping your temperature steady to delivering nutrition to your cells. It lubricates joints, delivers nutrition to every cell in your body, removes and filters out waste, and keeps your skin plump. With age, however, plums become prunes; similarly, the fluids in the human body gradually diminish. So during your perimenopausal years, the basic rule of thumb is this: Drink more water! Your skin looks drier and wrinkles appear more visible when you are dehydrated.

To keep hydrated during the menopausal transition and beyond, do the following:

- Aim for at least eight cups of water each day. Try for three cups before 10 a.m., three more cups by 4 p.m., and two more by 8 p.m. It's not so hard when you break it up!
- Fruits and vegetables are 70 to 97 percent water. For great nutrition and an edible source of water, eat a fruit or a vegetable at every meal and for most snacks.
- Have a soup or salad every day—a simple daily strategy to get more water.
- If you find that you forget to drink water, try keeping a pitcher with sixty-four ounces (eight cups) of water on your kitchen counter or on a conference table in your office along with a nice glass. Slice a whole orange or a couple of lemons into thin rings to add to the pitcher. It's colorful and pretty and may just get your attention to remind you to enjoy a glass.
- Keep eight mini eight-ounce bottles of flat or sparkling water in the refrigerator or lined up on a kitchen counter. Make it your daily goal to finish them.
- Don't forget teatime. Green tea, like all teas, is a great source of water. (So are vegetable juices and 100 percent fruit juices.)
- If you enjoy cold beverages, add ice. Ice is simply the solid form of water. Add a few cubes to freshly brewed green tea and store it in the refrigerator for an additional option. Take frozen blueberries and freeze them in ice cube trays with water for a fun way to get variety and to remind you to drink up.
- Keep a food or water journal to track your intake. Make it a game with a daily and a weekly goal. (I know this is a little "Type A," but it's worth a try.) If you're behind at the end of the week, don't try to make it all up in one day! Spread it out.

Don't Hold the Anchovies, Please

Eating a diet low in omega-3 can result in fatigue, dry skin, cracked nails, thin hair, and constipation. Consuming omega-3 from a variety of sources is essential. Fatty fish (like salmon, bluefish, mackerel, sardines, and anchovies) have a lot of omega-3—especially the component DHA, which is a building block for brain-tissue cells. Fish oil, egg yolks, and sea algae also contain omega-3. Those who shudder at the thought of fish should eat ground flaxseed and walnuts. There are lots of creative ways to get omega-3 in your diet.

Alisa's Fitness Tips

Looking good can be the best revenge (especially at your high school reunion), but feeling good—really good—is better than any form of revenge. There is no time in your life when feeling good is as important as it is at menopause. You will absolutely feel better if you do some form of exercise. This fact is beyond debate.

Although improving one's fitness is never easy, the effects of even moderate improvement are huge. Fifty really can be the new thirty. Exercise is one of the most inexpensive ways to treat aging. In fact, there are many fitness-related solutions for almost all menopausal symptoms. Here are some of the benefits of being fit.

Collagen production   Regular cardiovascular exercise helps your body establish an efficient basal metabolic rate. This can actually reset the cellular clock so that skin cells behave as though they belong to someone younger. Exercise slows or even appears to counteract the negative effects of estrogen depletion on the turnover of dead skin cells and the production of collagen and elastin.

According to yoga experts, forward-bending poses such as the bowing pose, the modified headstand, and the child pose increase blood supply to the underlying tissues of the face, giving skin a rosy glow and carrying the necessary nutrients for maximum collagen production.

Hot flashes   The complex mechanisms that trigger flushing and hot flashes during perimenopause aren't fully understood, but aerobic exercise helps regulate hormone production, which may explain why studies show that as little as twenty minutes of moderate exercise three times a week can significantly reduce the frequency and intensity of hot flashes.

Low abdominal breathing (see chapter 10) has also been shown to calm hot flashes. Combine programmed breathing with yoga or Tai Chi for a double dose of cool.

Dryness   Exercise stimulates the production of skin's natural moisturizing oils, which help to combat the decrease that occurs with estrogen depletion.

There is some scientific evidence behind the adage "Use it or lose it." For women experiencing menopausal vaginal dryness, more frequent sexual activity can actually increase natural lubrication.

In addition, cardiovascular exercise delivers nutrients efficiently to all the cells of your body, helping to keep them hydrated.

Insomnia   The insomnia that many women experience during perimenopause is triggered by what doctors call arousal, or overstimulation, of the nervous system. Along with the itchy, twitchy, sweaty tossing and turning, your mind becomes aroused as you lie awake thinking about how much you have to do the next day or how awful it is to be awake. Studies show that yoga, meditation, and other relaxation disciplines that focus on calm mindfulness can short-circuit the arousal before it becomes a self-fulfilling prophecy.

Moderate multimodal exercise—cardio combined with resistance training—has been shown to reduce insomnia in adults over sixty. Try moderate exercise to improve your sleep cycle, but make sure you complete your workout at least two hours before going to bed, or your body won't have time to return to a resting mode.

ASK DR. AVA

I saw an advertisement for a system of facial calisthenics, using a mouth device, that's supposed to completely eliminate wrinkles naturally. Can these exercises really firm aging skin?

Facial exercises unfortunately do very little to improve the appearance of aging skin. You might be able to get a short-term lifting effect by contracting the muscles of your face, but eventually gravity will have its way. Exercise doesn't tone facial muscles the way it does larger muscle groups. Facial wrinkling and sagging have much more to do with changes in the fat pads that support the skin than they do with muscle firmness. Furthermore, working your facial muscles may actually contribute to dynamic wrinkles—the kind of wrinkles that come from repeated movement over time.

A Fitness Story from Alisa

While training the *Extreme Makeover* participants, I discovered that many were suffering from uncomfortable symptoms of menopause. Improving their fitness not only dramatically helped their physiques and complexions, but the contestants also reported that their perimenopausal symptoms got better or in some cases vanished altogether. Exercise can increase the production of endorphins, the brain's own feel-good neurotransmitters. I saw relief in one participant from her menopausal-related feelings of depression and even extinguished another woman's debilitating perimenopausal insomnia.

Anxiety and mood swings   Studies have shown that exercise performed consistently for two weeks will noticeably improve your mood and offset feelings of depression and fatigue.

Working out at a gym is—not to put too fine a point on it—a great big snooze. Learning a new physical activity—tennis, swimming, salsa dancing—is not. Learning a new skill is an extremely effective way to overcome mild depression and anxiety. Your mind is programmed to pursue knowledge and accomplish goals, but brain scans show that there is little mental activity when depression sets in. Teaching yourself a new fitness skill can be a great way to turn that process around.

Work on your posture as a way to elevate your spirit. Start by holding your head high, walking tall, and sitting up straight. These postural adjustments send positive messages to your brain and to those around you.

Instead of medicating your midlife anxiety or depression with alcohol, which has both stimulant and sedative effects, use exercise. Both vigorous cardiovascular exercise and calming yoga release endorphins, the body's natural painkillers and mood lifters.

Skin Care Regimens for Menopausal Skin

OILY SKIN

MORNING REGIMEN

Step	Directions
Cleanse	Wash with a cleanser that contains glycolic acid.
Tone	If needed, apply oil-controlling toner.
Serum	To add more nutrients to your skin, apply serum to rejuvenate, firm, and address other concerns. Alpha-lipoic acid, coenzyme Q10 (ubiquinone), pomegranate, DMAE, lactic

acid, caffeine, copper peptide, ferulic acid, phytic acid, vitamin C, basil, grape seed extract, lutein, lycopene, green tea, ginseng, genistein, silymarin, vitamin E, human growth factor, resveratrol, acai berry, AHA, retinol, and apple stem cell address rejuvenation.

Eyes	Gently dot a small amount of cream around the eyes. Choose products with ingredients that address your areas of concern. Vitamin K, retinol, caffeine, vitamin C, yarrow, horse chestnut, and gingko biloba address dark circles. Haloxyl, caffeine, vitamin C, cucumber extract, green tea, and aloe vera address puffiness. Hyaluronic acid, silica, soy proteins, acai berry, aloe vera, seaweed extracts, GABA, and argireline address wrinkles, firmness, and elasticity.
Moisturize	Every day: Apply a small amount of a light, oil-free, non-comedogenic moisturizer with anti-oxidants. If you have additional skin care needs: Choose an oil-free moisturizer with ingredients designed to treat your specific skin care issues. Salicylic acid, benzoyl peroxide, retinol (for evening use only), azelaic acid, tea tree oil, phytic acid, and peppermint oil address oil production and breakouts. Green tea, calendula, cucumber, aloe vera, chamomile, thyme, willow herb, perilla leaf extract, feverfew, red clove, evening primrose oil, zinc, mallow, red algae, silymarin, ginger, lavender, azulene, and blue lotus address inflammation and irritation. Hydroquinone, mulberry extract, niacinamide, arbutin, bearberry extract, licorice extract, kojic acid, azelaic acid, and gallic acid address brown spots. AHA, alpha-lipoic acid, basil, coenzyme Q10, hyaluronic acid, pomegranate, DMAE, lactic acid, caffeine, copper peptide, ferulic acid, grape seed extract, phytic acid, vitamin C, vitamin E, retinol or retinoids (for evening use only), ursolic acid, silymarin, ginger, and ginseng address wrinkles.
Protect	Apply an oil-free, broad-spectrum, and non-comedogenic sunblock *every day*. *Note:* If your moisturizer contains a sunscreen of at least SPF 25 that blocks UVA and UVB rays, you don't need to add extra sunblock.

EVENING REGIMEN

Step	Directions
Cleanse	Wash with a cleanser that contains glycolic acid or tea tree oil.
Tone	If needed, gently wipe your face with toner or spray with facial water.
Serum	To add more nutrients to your skin, apply serum to rejuvenate, firm, and address other concerns. Alpha-lipoic acid, coenzyme Q10 (ubiquinone), pomegranate, DMAE, lactic acid, caffeine, copper peptide, ferulic acid, phytic acid, vitamin C, basil, grape seed extract, lutein, lycopene, green tea, ginseng, genistein, silymarin, vitamin E, resveratrol, acai berry, AHA, retinol, and apple stem cell address rejuvenation.

Eyes	Gently dot a small amount of cream around the eyes. Choose products with ingredients that address your areas of concern. Vitamin K, retinol, caffeine, vitamin C, yarrow, horse chestnut, and gingko biloba address dark circles. Haloxyl, caffeine, vitamin C, cucumber extract, green tea, and aloe vera address puffiness. Hyaluronic acid, silica, soy proteins, acai berry, aloe vera, seaweed extracts, GABA, and argireline address wrinkles, firmness, and elasticity.
Moisturize	Every evening: Apply a small amount of a moisturizing lotion with retinol. If you have additional skin care needs: Choose an oil-free moisturizer with ingredients designed to treat your specific skin care issues. Salicylic acid, benzoyl peroxide, retinol (for evening use only), azelaic acid, tea tree oil, phytic acid, and peppermint oil address oil production and breakouts. Green tea, calendula, cucumber, aloe vera, chamomile, thyme, willow herb, perilla leaf extract, feverfew, red clove, evening primrose oil, zinc, mallow, red algae, silymarin, ginger, lavender, azulene, and blue lotus address inflammation and irritation. Hydroquinone, mulberry extract, niacinamide, arbutin, bearberry extract, licorice extract, kojic acid, azelaic acid, and gallic acid address brown spots. AHA, alpha-lipoic acid, basil, coenzyme Q10, hyaluronic acid, pomegranate, DMAE, lactic acid, caffeine, copper peptide, ferulic acid, grape seed extract, phytic acid, vitamin C, vitamin E, retinol or retinoids (for evening use only), ursolic acid, silymarin, ginger, and ginseng address wrinkles.

INGREDIENTS TO AVOID

If your skin is excessively oily: Mineral oil, petrolatum, coconut oil

If your skin is highly sensitive: Lactic acid, glycolic acid, alpha-lipoic acid, acetic acid, benzoic acid, cinnamic acid, menthol, parabens, quaternium-15, vitamin C

If you have existing discoloration: Celery extract, lime extract, parsley extract, fig extract, carrot extract, bergamot oil, estradiol, genistein

If your skin is acne-prone: Butyl stearate, cinnamon oil, isostearyl isostearate, cocoa butter, jojoba oil, coconut oil, decyl oleate, myristyl myristate, myristyl propionate, octyl palminate, octyl stearate, peppermint oil, isopropyl stearate, isopropyl isostearate, myristate, palmitate

AT-HOME TREATMENTS

You can purchase over-the-counter masks and exfoliates for oily skin, or you can make your own (see chapter 11).

Masks	You can apply a mask once or twice a week to tighten the pores and temporarily reduce excessive oil production. Masks are also helpful in reducing inflammation from acne flares.

Exfoliation	As long as your skin is relatively calm, you can use a gentle exfoliating scrub once a week. If you are experiencing a flare-up of acne or excessive oil production, do not use *any* kind of scrub.

IN-OFFICE PROCEDURES

Peel   Microdermabrasion   Deep-cleansing facial   Laser treatment

Photo-dynamic therapy   Radio-frequency treatment

COMBINATION SKIN

MORNING REGIMEN

Step	Directions
Cleanse	Wash with a soap-free cleanser that contains polyhydroxy acid.
Tone	Gently wipe your face with a hydrating toner or spray with an antioxidant mist. You can use glycolic acid pads or oil-control gel on the T-zone, if needed.
Serum	To add more nutrients to your skin, apply serum to rejuvenate, firm, and address other concerns. Alpha-lipoic acid, coenzyme Q10 (ubiquinone), pomegranate, DMAE, lactic acid, caffeine, copper peptide, ferulic acid, phytic acid, vitamin C, basil, grape seed extract, lutein, lycopene, green tea, ginseng, genistein, silymarin, vitamin E, resveratrol, acai berry, AHA, retinol, and apple stem cell address rejuvenation.
Eyes	Gently dot a small amount of cream around the eyes. Choose products with ingredients that address your areas of concern. Vitamin K, retinol, caffeine, vitamin C, yarrow, horse chestnut, and gingko biloba address dark circles. Haloxyl, caffeine, vitamin C, cucumber extract, green tea, and aloe vera address puffiness. Hyaluronic acid, silica, soy proteins, acai berry, aloe vera, seaweed extracts, GABA, and argireline address wrinkles, firmness, and elasticity.

Moisturize	Every day:
	    Apply a small amount of moisturizer with antioxidants.
	If you have additional skin care needs:
	    Choose a moisturizer with ingredients designed to treat your specific skin care issues. Azelaic acid, salicylic acid, glycolic acid, retinol (for evening use only), tea tree oil, and zinc address oil production and breakouts. Hyaluronic acid, ceramide, olive oil, dexpanthenol (provitamin B_5), evening primrose oil, borage seed oil, colloidal oatmeal, apricot kernel oil, macadamia nut oil, safflower oil, and jojoba oil address hydration.

Niacinamide, kojic acid, mulberry extract, vitamin C, pine bark extract, strawberry begonia, and magnesium ascorbyl phosphate address brown spots. Aloe vera, green tea, calendula, cucumber, thyme, chamomile, willow herb, perilla leaf extract, feverfew, evening primrose oil, red clove, mirabilis, colloidal oatmeal, red algae, and zinc address irritation and inflammation. Caffeine, green tea extract, coenzyme Q10 (ubiquinone), carrot extract, rosemary, grape seed extract, genistein (soy), caffeine, copper peptide, ferulic acid, lutein, rosemary, basil, ginkgo biloba, and vitamin C address wrinkles. Azelaic acid, salicylic acid, retinol (for evening use only), tea tree oil, and zinc address acne flares.

Protect	Apply broad-spectrum sunblock *every day*. *Note:* If your moisturizer contains a sunscreen of at least SPF 25 that blocks UVA and UVB rays, you don't need to add extra sunblock.

EVENING REGIMEN

Step	*Directions*
Cleanse	Wash your face with a cleanser that contains a low percentage of glycolic acid.
Tone	Gently wipe your face with hydrating toner. You can use glycolic acid pads on the T-zone, if needed.
Serum	To add more nutrients to your skin, apply serum to rejuvenate, firm, and address other concerns. Alpha-lipoic acid, coenzyme Q10 (ubiquinone), pomegranate, DMAE, lactic acid, caffeine, copper peptide, ferulic acid, phytic acid, vitamin C, basil, grape seed extract, lutein, lycopene, green tea, ginseng, genistein, silymarin, vitamin E, resveratrol, acai berry, AHA, retinol, and apple stem cell address rejuvenation.
Eyes	Gently dot a small amount of cream around the eyes. Choose products with ingredients that address your areas of concern. Vitamin K, retinol, caffeine, vitamin C, yarrow, horse chestnut, and gingko biloba address dark circles. Haloxyl, caffeine, vitamin C, cucumber extract, green tea, and aloe vera address puffiness. Hyaluronic acid, silica, soy proteins, acai berry, aloe vera, seaweed extracts, GABA, and argireline address wrinkles, firmness, and elasticity.
Moisturize	Every evening: Apply a small amount of a moisturizing lotion with retinol. If you have additional skin care needs: Choose an oil-free moisturizer with ingredients designed to treat your specific skin care issues. Azelaic acid, salicylic acid, glycolic acid, retinol (for evening use only), tea tree oil, and zinc address oil production and breakouts. Hyaluronic acid, ceramide, olive oil, dexpanthenol (provitamin B_5), evening primrose oil, borage seed oil, colloidal oatmeal, apricot kernel oil, macadamia nut oil, safflower oil, and jojoba oil address hydration. Niacinamide, kojic acid, mulberry extract, vitamin C, pine bark extract, strawberry begonia, and magnesium ascorbyl phosphate address brown spots. Aloe vera, green tea,

calendula, cucumber, thyme, chamomile, willow herb, perilla leaf extract, feverfew, evening primrose oil, red clove, mirabilis, colloidal oatmeal, red algae, and zinc address irritation and inflammation. Caffeine, green tea extract, coenzyme Q10 (ubiquinone), carrot extract, rosemary, grape seed extract, genistein (soy), caffeine, copper peptide, ferulic acid, lutein, rosemary, basil, ginkgo biloba, and vitamin C address wrinkles. Azelaic acid, salicylic acid, retinol (for evening use only), tea tree oil, and zinc address acne flares.

INGREDIENTS TO AVOID

If your skin is excessively oily: Mineral oil, petrolatum, coconut oil

If your skin is highly sensitive: Lactic acid, glycolic acid, alpha-lipoic acid, acetic acid, benzoic acid, cinnamic acid, menthol, parabens, quaternium-15, vitamin C

If you have existing discoloration: Celery extract, lime extract, parsley extract, fig extract, carrot extract, bergamot oil, estradiol, genistein

If your skin is acne-prone: Butyl stearate, cinnamon oil, isostearyl isostearate, cocoa butter, jojoba oil, coconut oil, decyl oleate, myristyl myristate, myristyl propionate, octyl palminate, octyl stearate, peppermint oil, isopropyl stearate, isopropyl isostearate, myristate, palmitate

AT-HOME TREATMENTS

You can purchase over-the-counter masks and exfoliates for combination skin, or you can make your own (see chapter 11).

Masks	Your skin will benefit from using a mask once or twice a week to deliver hydration and high concentrations of nutrients.
Exfoliation	To remove the top layer of dead skin cells, you may use a fine-textured scrub to exfoliate once a week. Don't exfoliate if you have very sensitive skin or if your acne medication causes irritation.

IN-OFFICE PROCEDURES

Peel	Microdermabrasion	Cleansing and hydrating facial treatment
Laser treatment	Radio-frequency treatment	

DRY SKIN

MORNING REGIMEN

Step	Directions
Cleanse	Wash with a gentle, soothing nonfoaming cleanser or use cold cream.

Tone	Mist your face with antioxidant spray and follow quickly with the application of a hydrating serum.
Serum	To add more nutrients to your skin, apply serum to rejuvenate, firm, and address other concerns. Alpha-lipoic acid, coenzyme Q10 (ubiquinone), pomegranate, DMAE, lactic acid, caffeine, copper peptide, ferulic acid, phytic acid, vitamin C, basil, grape seed extract, lutein, lycopene, green tea, ginseng, genistein, silymarin, vitamin E, resveratrol, acai berry, AHA, retinol, and apple stem cell address rejuvenation.
Eyes	Gently dot a small amount of cream around the eyes. Choose products with ingredients that address your areas of concern. Vitamin K, caffeine, vitamin C, yarrow, horse chestnut, and gingko biloba address dark circles. Haloxyl, caffeine, vitamin C, cucumber extract, green tea, and aloe vera address puffiness. Hyaluronic acid, silica, soy proteins, acai berry, aloe vera, seaweed extracts, GABA, retinol, and argireline address wrinkles, firmness, and elasticity.

Moisturize	Every day:
	    Apply moisturizer while your skin is still damp from the hydrating serum.
	If you have additional skin care needs:
	    Choose a moisturizer with ingredients designed to treat your specific skin care issues. Ceramides, borage seed oil, canola oil, apricot kernel oil, cocoa butter (don't use if you have acne), dexpanthenol, olive oil, glycerin, evening primrose oil, jojoba oil, macadamia nut oil, shea butter, safflower oil, colloidal oatmeal, dimethicone, lanolin (don't use if you have acne), and pumpkinseed oil address hydration. Green tea, calendula, cucumber, aloe vera, chamomile, feverfew, colloidal oatmeal, aloe vera, and thyme address irritation and inflammation. Arbutin, bearberry, coconut palm, cucumber extract, willow herb, gallic acid, hydroquinone, kojic acid, retinol (for evening use only), vitamin C, mulberry extract, and pycnogenol (pine bark extract) address brown spots. AHA, basil, lutein, lycopene, citric acid, lactic acid, phytic acid, polyhydroxy acid, retinol (for evening use only), carrot extract, rosemary, grape seed extract, genistein, caffeine, copper peptide, ferulic acid, and DMAE address wrinkles. Salicylic acid, azelaic acid, benzoyl peroxide, retinol (for evening use only), and tea tree oil address acne flares (precede with moisturizer if skin is very dry).

Protect	Apply broad-spectrum sunblock *every day.* *Note:* If your moisturizer contains a sunscreen of at least SPF 25 that blocks UVA and UVB rays, you don't need to add extra sunblock.

EVENING REGIMEN

Step	Directions
Cleanse	Wash your face with a soap-free cleanser that contains calendula, chamomile, or other soothing ingredients.

Tone	Mist your face with facial rose water or a hydrating toner.
Serum	To add more nutrients to your skin, apply serum to rejuvenate, firm, and address other concerns. Alpha-lipoic acid, coenzyme Q10 (ubiquinone), pomegranate, DMAE, lactic acid, caffeine, copper peptide, ferulic acid, phytic acid, vitamin C, basil, grape seed extract, lutein, lycopene, green tea, ginseng, genistein, silymarin, vitamin E, resveratrol, acai berry, AHA, retinol, and apple stem cell address rejuvenation.
Eyes	Gently dot a small amount of cream around the eyes. Choose products with ingredients that address your areas of concern. Vitamin K, retinol, caffeine, vitamin C, yarrow, horse chestnut, and gingko biloba address dark circles. Haloxyl, caffeine, vitamin C, cucumber extract, green tea, and aloe vera address puffiness. Hyaluronic acid, silica, soy proteins, acai berry, aloe vera, seaweed extracts, GABA, and argireline address wrinkles, firmness, and elasticity.
Moisturize	Every evening: While your skin is still damp, apply a moisturizer that contains moisture-locking ingredients like ceramides and peptides. If you have additional skin care needs: Choose a moisturizer with ingredients designed to treat your specific skin care issues. Ceramides, borage seed oil, canola oil, apricot kernel oil, cocoa butter (don't use if you have acne), dexpanthenol, olive oil, glycerin, evening primrose oil, jojoba oil, macadamia nut oil, shea butter, safflower oil, colloidal oatmeal, dimethicone, lanolin (don't use if you have acne), and pumpkinseed oil address hydration. Green tea, calendula, cucumber, aloe vera, chamomile, feverfew, colloidal oatmeal, aloe vera, and thyme address irritation and inflammation. Arbutin, bearberry, coconut palm, cucumber extract, willow herb, gallic acid, hydroquinone, kojic acid, retinol (for evening use only), vitamin C, mulberry extract, and pycnogenol (pine bark extract) address brown spots. AHA, basil, lutein, lycopene, citric acid, lactic acid, phytic acid, polyhydroxy acid, retinol (for evening use only), carrot extract, rosemary, grape seed extract, genistein, caffeine, copper peptide, ferulic acid, and DMAE address wrinkles. Salicylic acid, azelaic acid, benzoyl peroxide, retinol (for evening use only), and tea tree oil address acne flares (precede with moisturizer if skin is very dry).

INGREDIENTS TO AVOID

If your skin is highly sensitive: Alcohol, lactic acid, glycolic acid, alpha-lipoic acid, acetic acid, benzoyl acid, cinnamic acid, polyhydroxy acid, phytic acid, vitamin C

If you have existing discoloration: Estradiol, estrogen, genistein, dandelion, geranium, jasmine, lavender, lemongrass, lemon oil, neroli oil, rose oil, tea tree oil, sandalwood

If your skin is acne-prone: Cinnamon oil, isotearyl isostearate, cocoa butter, coconut oil, peppermint oil, isopropyl myristate, isopropyl isostearate

AT-HOME TREATMENTS

You can purchase over-the-counter mask and exfoliates for dry skin, or you can make your own (see chapter 11).

Masks	Masks can hydrate, reduce irritation, and be very soothing. Make sure when you buy an over-the-counter mask that it is specifically made for sensitive skin and contains none of the chemicals or ingredients listed above. If you have an acne flare or rosacea, talk to your doctor before using a mask on your face or your body.
Exfoliation	Use very gentle facial exfoliates. Homemade scrubs are a good option. Make sure that the product doesn't contain any fragrance or other chemicals. If your skin is very sensitive, you can use dry oatmeal to exfoliate. Do not use any peels or other microdermabrasion kits.

IN-OFFICE PROCEDURES

Cleansing and hydrating facial treatment   Laser treatment   Radio-frequency treatment

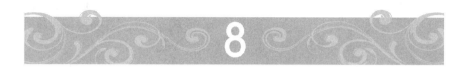

Adult Acne

HEALING YOUR SKIN

A well-known actress came to see me, disguising her lovely face under a large floppy hat to avoid being noticed. It turned out that the hat served two purposes: it hid her famous features *and* a breakout of adult acne.

"What am I going to do about my skin?" she asked me. "I keep getting pimples, and I have to start filming a hot romantic comedy with a lot of close-ups. When we go in for a kiss, a big zit on my chin will look gigantic on a twenty-foot movie screen!"

We both shuddered and then laughed. I told her what I tell all the women who come to me for treatment of their adult acne: you are not alone, and we can heal your skin.

Many of my patients are confused about the onset of acne well past their teenage years: "Why is it happening now? Aren't I too old? Where is the justice in having acne and wrinkles at the same time?" There is no justice! According to the *British Journal of Dermatology*, the incidence of acne is on the rise, along with the average age of acne sufferers. I've certainly seen this trend in my own practice.

There are two main reasons: changes in our diet and exercise patterns as well as the increased stress we endure every day. By trading fresh food for easy-to-prepare processed foods, we inadvertently ingest low-quality nutrients that don't support our skin. Our stress levels go through the roof as we try to juggle so many responsibilities—parent, employee, spouse, caretaker—all at once.

You may not have to fret about showing your face on a giant movie screen, but your face is still your calling card. If your skin is unhealthy or damaged and you don't like how you look, it can affect almost every other aspect of your life.

I find this to be especially true for my patients who suffer from adult acne. "My boss told me to go home because my face looked like a pizza," my patient Linda told me. She never wanted to hear those words again; she wanted to feel more confident around her family and to be able to leave her house without spending hours putting on cover-up. But most importantly, Linda wanted to stop spending so much time *thinking* about her skin. Working together, we developed a treatment plan that included a series of laser treatments, peels, and an at-home regimen that specifically addressed her adult acne.

In this chapter, you will learn:

- What adult acne looks like
- The role stress, hormones, and medication play in the formation of adult acne
- Adult acne imitators
- Complications of adult acne
- How to heal your skin: The Dr. Ava Plan
- Adult acne treatment options
- Nutrition and fitness tips for better-looking skin
- Skin care regimens for adult acne

Adult Acne versus Teen Acne

What does adult acne look like, and how does it differ from teenage break-outs? Adult acne may take a different form than teen acne. It can occur with fewer, larger pustules and more blackheads or small reddish bumps. It may be limited to redness and a feeling of tightness under the skin, or flare into fiery, deep-seated cysts. You may also have to deal with new outbreaks on skin already scarred from earlier acne bouts. If you have a dark skin tone, your biggest acne complaint may not be blemishes themselves but discoloration and scarring that occur when the blemish subsides.

The blemish you see is only the tip of the adult acne iceberg. Blackheads, whiteheads, pimples, and cysts are the result of a process that begins weeks before they appear. That time lag is important to remember when you're trying to get a handle on what triggers your outbreaks and keeps them coming, like waves to the seashore. And it's also crucial for designing an effective treatment plan.

Acne Formation

Like teen acne, adult acne forms in the pilosebaceous unit, tiny little hair oil glands that stud most of our skin. These units are essential to the vitality of the skin, but when they malfunction, acne can form. In acne,

	Adult Acne	Teen Acne
Location	Along the hairline, chin, neck	Forehead, nose, cheeks, back
Onset	Late twenties to fifties, may fluctuate with menstrual cycle	Puberty
Cause	Stress, hormonal changes, diet	Genetics, diet
Sequelae	Brown spots, discoloration, wrinkles	Depressed or pitted scars
Family history	No	Yes
Duration	Sporadic, may end at menopause	Two to fifteen years

DR. AVA'S MYTH BREAKER

The myth: Acne is caused by a buildup of dirt, and scrubbing your face is the only way to get rid of it.

The truth: Acne is not caused by grime, and your face is not a skillet that needs to be scrubbed clean. Using harsh cleansers and being too rough on your skin will actually make your acne worse by irritating the skin, possibly leaving it open to infection, and certainly causing more inflammation.

sebum production and keratinization, or epidermal cell production, ramp up, but the natural sloughing process slows down. *P. acnes*, bacteria normally found on the skin, proliferate in the follicle, chewing up the sebum.

The by-products of this sebum digestion induce an inflammatory reaction by the body. When your body gets the inflammatory alarm, it sends help rushing to the battleground. Unfortunately, there's collateral damage. The white blood cells (neutrophils) that arrive to mop up the bacterial invasion release enzymes that can damage or rupture the wall of the follicle, creating the red bump we affectionately know as a pimple. These inflammatory mediators and enzymes can also chew up your collagen, leading to scarring and the deepening of your wrinkles, as well as activating the melanin system, which causes the formation of a brown mark when the dreaded pimple finally goes away.

The Adult Acne Guilty Parties

What triggers acne again in your adult years or brings it on for the first time? Consider my patient Amanda. She was thirty-two years old, working as a high-powered attorney in a Beverly Hills firm, married to a television executive, and raising a young child when she first came to me for treatment of her acne.

"I had mild acne on my cheeks, but that has been gone for years," she told me. "Now I am breaking out on my jawline, neck, and upper back, and when it goes away I am left with brown spots. What is going on?"

Amanda had all the classic features of adult acne. Her acne was located in areas that are common for adult acne breakouts. The acne was leaving behind brown spots after it cleared. She lived a very stressful lifestyle, one of the three main contributors to the onset of adult acne. The other two factors are hormonal fluctuations and medication use. You may be affected by one, two, or all three at the same time.

Stress

To put it simply: As teenagers, acne gives us stress. As adults, stress gives us acne.

The skin performs its many assigned functions quietly when there is peace in the land. But when disruptions occur (such as a lack of sleep because we have so many responsibilities), the very hormone that is being produced to allow the body to function at peak performance can backfire, wreaking havoc on the skin. (I've seen many actors with persistent acne because they constantly need to deliver peak performances.)

We are designed to rise to the occasion, so to speak. When faced with danger, we need to be able to bolt away. Our adrenal glands pump out cortisol to help us escape but also to help us deliver a peak performance. New research shows that sebaceous glands can act as their own independent endocrine organs. This means that your brain can directly stimulate sebaceous activity by the release of a corticotrophin-releasing hormone, which rises during stress.

Cortisol and other adrenal steroids can stimulate the sebaceous glands, resulting in acne flare-ups. Cortisol is going to pump any time you are experiencing a stressful moment, regardless of whether you've just read a hostile text message from your mother-in-law, you've just won the lottery, or you're an Olympic athlete poised at the starting gate of a race. In addition, when we are stressed out, we crave junk food and carbohydrates—another response to the rise in cortisol. This can trigger or worsen acne breakouts.

There's a kind of feedback loop that operates with acne. Your stress triggers a breakout, and then

---

DR. AVA'S MYTH BREAKERS

The myth: Working up a sweat will make your acne worse.

The truth: Acne does not begin in sweat glands. Although sweat may irritate skin that has been made dry by acne treatment, sweat in itself won't cause breakouts. Exercise can actually help, because it is a great stress reliever. After your workout, clean your skin gently, pat dry, and apply moisturizer. Pay special attention to cleaning and drying the areas where sweat and sebum can build up: under bike helmets, chin guards, and bike shorts. Localized treatment may be necessary to clear up these areas.

The myth: Sunbathing and tanning will clear up your acne.

The truth: It's true that *P. acnes*, the bacteria that is one trigger of inflammatory lesions, is destroyed by sunlight. Nevertheless, the risks of unprotected exposure to ultraviolet radiation—whether from the sun's rays or a tanning bed— far outweigh any theoretical benefit. Most acne treatments, whether topical, oral, or mechanical, also make your skin more sensitive to UV radiation. So use a good, nongreasy sunblock and protect yourself from premature aging by the sun.

ASK DR. AVA

I'm a woman in my twenties with severe acne. My period has always been irregular, but now it's stopped completely, and I'm starting to notice hair growth on my face while the hair on my head is thinning. What is happening to me?

At your age, your combination of symptoms—acne, scalp hair loss, facial hair growth, and amenorrhea (not having your period)— may mean that you have a condition known as polycystic ovary syndrome (PCOS), especially if you are overweight. Because PCOS can affect your fertility and put you at risk for heart disease and other illnesses, see your health care professional as soon as possible. Your doctor can also look for other causes for your symptoms, which include thyroid disease or an androgen-producing tumor.

your breakout triggers more stress. The goal is to break the cycle by treating both the acne and the stress. For example, one of my patients, who is a very successful talent agent, mother, wife, *and* movie producer, has treated her acne with topical skin care, adjusted her diet, and calmed her stress through acupuncture and an exercise program.

Hormonal Fluctuations

Hormones are behind the majority of adult acne breakouts. If you're a woman who is genetically prone to acne, you may notice that your breakouts coincide with the premenstrual part of your cycle, when estrogen levels drop. This leaves the androgens produced by the ovaries, like testosterone, unopposed to stimulate the sebaceous gland, which thereby pumps up oil secretions.

The hormonal shifts around pregnancy, childbirth, and breastfeeding, as well as menopause, can be accompanied by new or recurring acne. (The skin implications of pregnancy and menopause are covered in separate chapters.) You may also notice that your breakouts coincide with your weekly conference with your boss—in other words, from the hormones associated with stress.

Medication Use

In some cases, your acne may be a side effect of a medication. When you seek treatment for acne, it's important to mention any drugs you are taking. The following drugs are most often associated with new or worsened acne flares:

- Oral or injected prescription steroids for asthma, endocrine, and other respiratory disorders

- Antiseizure medications that are prescribed for epilepsy
- Lithium, used in the treatment of bipolar disorder
- Certain medications that contain bromides or iodides
- Antabuse, prescribed in the treatment of alcoholism
- Oral contraceptives—discontinuing use or switching from one brand to another
- Anabolic steroids, like those used illegally by athletes and bodybuilders

The good news is that acne caused by medication use will clear up once you stop taking the medication. If you have to take one of these medications for a long time, you'll need to work with your health care team to develop an effective skin care regimen.

Adult acne can also appear anywhere you apply repeated or extended pressure on your skin. Resting your chin on your hand while

DR. AVA'S MYTH BREAKER

The myth: It's okay to pop your pimples as long as you do it the right way.

The truth: There's absolutely no right way to pop or otherwise drain a pimple or blemish. Scratching, poking, and popping blemishes significantly increase the risk of infection and scarring. A health care professional can perform extractions under sterile conditions.

Acne Imitators

A complete discussion of rashes that look like acne but aren't is beyond the scope of this book, but be aware that there are several skin conditions that mimic adult acne:

Contact dermatitis   Redness or bumps may be a sign that you're sensitive to something that you're putting on your skin. Soaps, cleansers, skin care products, makeup, aftershave, fragrances, hair care products, and even your laundry detergent can cause these bumps.

Folliculitis   Reddened bumps or pimples that occur in places where you frequently shave, pluck, or wax may be the sign of an ingrown hair or an irritation or infection in the hair follicle.

Miliaria   Popularly known as *heat rash* or *prickly heat*, miliaria occurs when the pores of the sweat glands are blocked with dead skin cells.

Rosacea   Rosacea may appear as flushing, facial swelling, dilated blood vessels, and disfiguration of the nose.

you work, pressing your cell phone against your chin, or wearing tight clothing can cause acne. No one understands why this happens, but if it does, be conscious of touching your face; switch to a headset, or buy the next size up in bike shorts. (Surveys show that we touch our faces ten to twelve times an hour.)

Complications from Adult Acne

There are two common complications from adult acne: post-inflammatory hyperpigmentation (PIH) and scarring. PIH is the most common form of acne-related skin discoloration and occurs when excess pigment (melanin) is produced and deposited in the cells of the epidermis as a response to acne inflammation. This results in brownish spots with blurred edges, most often occurring at the site of a previous blemish. This happens more frequently in adult acne and particularly in people with skin of color, who have more pigment in their skin.

These marks can persist for many months and may not resolve on their own. Patients often call these brown spots "acne scars," but they are not scars. A true acne scar is a geographical change in the landscape of the skin that appears as a shallow indentation or a small, deep "stab" scar called an ice-pick scar or a raised keloidal scar. In fact, true acne scars can take many shapes, and a person can have more than one type on his or her face. It is not understood why some people with acne develop severe scarring but others remain unmarked. Geographical changes in the skin can be extremely difficult to cover with makeup and require intervention with lasers, injectables, or surgery to eliminate them.

The Shamban Scale

You know you have acne. Now you want to know how to get rid of it. Although there is no "cure" for acne, there are a wide variety of effective treatment options. In fact, acne treatment has advanced a very long way in a fairly short time, and continues to do so. There is no reason to feel hopeless about your persistent acne or because treatments failed in the past. I urge you to see a dermatologist today. There is real help for managing adult acne and for significantly revising acne scarring.

I'll admit, it's not always simple. Acne manifests in an amazingly complex range of symptoms. It is complicated by stress, hormonal changes, and other health issues. The way skin responds to acne treatment is also complex and often idiosyncratic—what works for you may not work for someone else. What works for you may not even work for you all the time. It's as though acne is a different condition for everyone who has it.

Older models for classifying acne used to reflect this level of complexity. There were numerous scales for grading severity, often requiring dizzying calculations like counting individual blemishes. These differing systems made it difficult to compare the success of treatment programs. Recently I helped develop a new, simpler scale for classifying the severity of acne, based on in-office observation and grading of the three most common treatment concerns: (1) the acne itself, (2) acne scarring, and (3) pigmentation or discoloration. Each patient is assigned a score from zero to three in each of these three categories, and a personalized treatment plan is developed based on that score.

For example, if you came to see me with lots of blackheads and whiteheads but no inflammatory lesions, and with a significant degree of scarring from past outbreaks but no discoloration, your acne would be rated A1–S2–P0 on the Shamban Scale. We would then work together to develop a treatment plan to clear your skin of current blemishes and to minimize scars.

THE SHAMBAN SCALE

Acne (A)	Acne Scarring (S)	Pigmentation (P)
0 None	0 None	0 None
1 Mild	1 Mild	1 Mild
2 Moderate	2 Moderate	2 Moderate
3 Severe	3 Severe	3 Severe

The Adult Acne Plan of Action

Every great military campaign begins with a great commander. In the battle against adult acne, this can be you! Fortunately, there are a wide variety of effective treatment options that you can do at home. These include over-the-counter topical acne preparations ranging from masks to skin care regimens to acne-zapping light devices.

Without a doubt, as with any self-improvement program, getting results requires commitment, time, and patience. Sometimes you will need in-office treatment by a dermatologist. In most instances, however, a coordinated program that addresses your skin by incorporating a total-body health approach through skin care, fitness, and a balanced diet will lead to a clearer complexion along with a better frame of mind and a healthier you.

Healing Your Adult Acne: The Dr. Ava Plan

We all have a routine that we do every morning to get ready for our day. We brush our teeth, fix our hair, and choose our clothes, yet we often neglect the most important accessory we own: our faces. First and foremost, good skin requires consistency. That means washing your face every morning and evening and applying your anti-acne medication in a sophisticated fashion. Never spot-treat only; always cover your entire face. Not only are you are clearing up your acne, you are also repairing your wrinkles and fighting the breakouts you don't see yet.

The program I have designed will not only treat your active acne, it will also address the discoloration associated with adult acne as well as the annoying early lines and wrinkles that are adult acne's bedside companions.

Phase 1: Cleanse

Proper cleansing of your skin is a lot like the dilemma of Goldilocks in search of the perfect porridge. Too much cleansing of the skin can be just as damaging as too little cleansing; it has to be done "just right." The sebum is the body's self-made moisturizer. It also protects you from bacteria such as MRSA, viruses (like those that cause warts), and fungi. Removing too much sebum from the surface of the skin will not lower its production and will either overdry the skin, leaving more dry skin cells to mix with existing sebum, which can then clog pores, or cause a reflex oiliness. If the skin is not adequately cleansed, dirt and bacteria will cling to the sebum, which is sticky by nature, and contribute to acne formation.

Although salicylic acid doesn't slow down oil production or kill bacteria, it is an ideal ingredient in an over-the-counter acne-cleansing preparation because of its ability to clear away the buildup of dead skin cells and unclog pores. Preparations that contain salicylic acid are particularly useful in controlling blackheads and whiteheads. Because it's an anti-inflammatory (in the form of aspirin, it lowers a fever and relieves pain), salicylic acid may also fight redness. Like most acne-fighting ingredients, it can be drying or irritating, so look for a product with a 2 percent concentration. Sometimes less is more, especially when it comes to acne.

To get the most benefit from your salicylic acid cleanser:

1. Wet your skin.
2. Put a dollop of the cleanser in the palm of one hand or onto a soft, clean washcloth.
3. Apply to the entire affected area, which may include not only your face but also your upper neck, back, and chest. Avoid the undereye area.
4. Brush your teeth, check your text messages, or update your Facebook page so that the product can stay on your skin for a few minutes.
5. Rinse with copious amounts of warm (not hot) water.

Phase 2: Kill Bacteria

Now that your skin has been cleansed, you need to apply a topical acne treatment to kill the acne culprit, *P. acnes.*

The workhorse of over-the-counter acne treatments, benzoyl peroxide, attacks *P. acnes* bacteria and speeds up the removal of dead skin cells. Because it is available without a prescription as a lotion or a gel, benzoyl peroxide has been the mainstay of acne treatment. The treatment must be continued even after flare-ups have subsided. Before using benzoyl peroxide, be sure to patch-test it on the inside of your arm to make sure you don't have an allergy.

To get the most benefit out of benzoyl peroxide:

1. Choose a product with 2.5 to 5 percent strength in a delivery form that is designed to reduce irritation, such as microsponge or extended release.
2. Apply a very thin layer, just enough to cover the entire affected area.
3. Lightly blot off any excess with a clean white washcloth. (It will bleach a colored washcloth.)

Phase 3: Reduce Inflammation

Adult acne can be highly inflammatory, leaving red welts on your skin. Reducing the inflammation is best done with a combination approach, using botanically derived antioxidants as well as members of the alpha-hydroxy family. These antioxidants act directly to reduce the production of the cell-mediated cytokines that are released at different stages of acne-genesis. They also capture free radicals.

Lactic acid and glycolic acid are the two alpha-hydroxy acids (AHAs) most commonly found in over-the-counter acne preparations. As exfoliants, they strip the skin of dead cells, giving a smooth texture to the skin and allowing it to look more luminous. They also draw moisture to the surface, which can alleviate the drying effects of other acne medications. In addition, AHAs are able to dissolve sebaceous plugs inside closed pores.

Next to retinoic acid, AHAs are possibly the most versatile of active skin ingredients. By exfoliating and loosening clogged pores, they enable the penetration of acne medication. They increase the production of complex sugars in the skin (the glycosaminoglycans), plump the skin, and can even out the pigment layer.

There are numerous antioxidants available in serums, lotions, creams, and mists. You can also make your own at-home version. Choose a vehicle that is compatible with your skin type. For example, a serum is best for dry skin, whereas a mist is ideal for oily skin. Antioxidants such as vitamin C have been shown to stimulate collagen production, which makes them an ideal choice for adults who suffer from both acne and signs of aging such as lines and wrinkles.

To get the most benefit out of AHAs and antioxidants:

1. Apply a thin layer of a serum or a lotion that contains an antioxidant (see the skin care regimes at the end of this chapter) or spray an antioxidant mist over the entire affected area.
2. Apply a thin layer of a low-strength AHA (8 to 10 percent) to the entire affected area.
3. Apply a moisturizer, if needed.

Phase 4: Treat Resistant Acne, Brown Spots, and Wrinkles

If four weeks have passed and you don't see any improvement in your acne or you have been left with discoloration from previous acne blemishes, you need to try a retinol. Retinols will also address the wrinkles that you are certain weren't there a month ago.

Vitamin A derivatives   At prescription levels, vitamin A derivatives are powerful anti-acne weapons, normalizing the process of skin-cell turnover and development. At over-the-counter levels, retinoids are still effective, but vitamin A in the form of retinol is highly unstable, and the concentrations are difficult to maintain in the presence of light and air. Unless vitamin A is listed as one of the top five ingredients and the retinol is in an airtight opaque bottle, the product is unlikely to be effective.

Retinoids bring your skin cells' turnover cycle back into alignment, preventing the buildup of sticky dead cells in the hair follicles and promoting the growth of healthy cells that slough off naturally. Some early retinoid formulations were extremely irritating, causing intense redness and burning, while the newer preparations do not.

Most likely, you'll still notice some stinging, redness, and peeling, particularly in the early days of treatment. Stick with it, and you'll see results. I've seen the power of retinoids work an extreme makeover on the skin, and I believe that anyone with resistant acne in mature skin—no matter what type or degree of severity—should be treated with some form of topical retinoid.

To get the best results when using a retinoid:

1. Use a nondetergent facial cleanser.
2. Start with a low percentage and work up as your skin begins to respond and becomes more tolerant of the irritating effects.
3. Always apply a sunscreen of at least SPF 25.
4. Moisturize.
5. Exercise caution. Discuss any retinoid treatment with your doctor if you are pregnant or breast-feeding or if you have a darker skin tone.
6. Expect a flare. About two or three weeks into retinoid treatment, you may see an acne eruption. That's the result of all those buried microcomedones being pushed to the surface as the retinoid works to normalize skin-cell turnover and clear the pores.
7. Expect to look younger. The retinoids used to control your adult acne will also have a noticeable anti-aging effect on your skin.

Sulfur   Sulfur has been used for centuries to fight infection and soften scaly skin. It was one of the earliest anti-acne drugs. Combined with resorcinol—an ingredient that strips the skin of dead cells—it is still used in a number of spot treatments. Avoid resorcinol if you have darker skin tones, because it can be discoloring. Some fair-skinned people find sulfur less irritating than benzoyl peroxide.

Alcohol, often combined with acetone   Normally found in cleansers and toners, alcohol and acetone are intended to remove extra oil and make your skin feel cleaner. There are specific types of alcohol products that are more beneficial to the skin than others. Alcohol is a mild disinfectant, and acetone is a degreaser. If your skin is dry or if you're over forty, you may find these products too drying or irritating. Use witch hazel if you like the feeling of a bracing but mild toner.

Herbal or "natural" ingredients   A number of over-the-counter acne products include botanical essences, herbs, and other so-called natural ingredients. On their own, they have not been definitively shown to fight acne, although some do have antioxidant or antibacterial properties. They may be added for extra soothing or, if fragrant, aromatherapeutic purposes.

You'll usually find natural ingredients listed last on the label, which means that they're present only in trace amounts. If you have plant-based allergies such as hay fever, herbal ingredients may cause a sensitivity reaction and you should test them on your arm before applying to your face.

Moving the Doctor's Office Home

With advances in technology, part of the dermatology office has been moved into the home. You can now do a fairly effective peel and microdermabrasion, use a handheld light-based or thermal device, or give yourself a botanical anti-acne, anti-inflammatory mask. Be attuned to your skin's needs and don't overdo it, because there is the potential to damage your skin.

Microdermabrasion   Microdermabrasion devices remove the outermost layer of dry, dead skin cells. This intense exfoliation prevents the pores from being clogged by the buildup of these dead cells so your acne medication can penetrate to where it's needed most and remove one of the causes of acne.

Particularly for the adult acne population, microdermabrasion can reduce signs of UV damage such as bumpy texture, brown spots (lentigo), and fine lines. Caution must be exercised when using this with a particularly intense skin care regimen because of potential irritation. People with rosacea, cystic acne, or other medical skin conditions should always consult their dermatologists before using microdermabrasion devices. These devices can be used once a week (brand names: *Crystalift*, *Timepeel*, *Natural Diamond*, *Sylvan home microdermabrasion machine*, *Nutra Luxe Microdermasion*).

Sonic Skin Cleansing   Sonic technology (the same technology that's behind cleaning your teeth) is a gentle but effective deep-cleansing system that uses an oscillating brush to loosen dirt and oil, clear the pores, and stimulate the skin through a micromassage action. This device can be extremely effective in cleaning oily skin without irritation and cleaning the skin on the back, which can be difficult to properly cleanse. Another advantage is that the brush can be used on all skin types twice a day with any nonabrasive cleanser (brand name: *Clarisonic*).

Handheld thermal devices   Cleared by the FDA for the treatment of mild to moderate acne, handheld thermal devices work by delivering a precisely controlled dosage of heat to a pimple through a metal pad. This causes the bacteria to self-destruct through a heat-shock response. A pimple can clear up with two or three treatments in a twenty-four-hour period. The drawback is that it is spot treatment only, can be used only for existing pimples, and does not prevent the formation of new ones (brand names: *Zeno, ThermaClear, no!no! Skin Acne Treatment System*).

Blue light and light-emitting diode treatments   Light-emitting diodes, a NASA-developed technology, have been shown to be effective in the treatment of mild to moderate acne. The blue light destroys bacteria while simultaneously addressing inflammation. It is nonthermal and nonablative (see chapter 7) and requires no downtime. These devices address existing breakouts and decrease the formation of new pimples. The only disadvantage is the amount of time required for treatment: up to twenty minutes. One system has an exchangeable head with a red light, which has been shown to stimulate collagen formation (brand names: *Evis MD, Tanda Clear Acne Light Therapy, Tria Skin Clarifying System, ANSR*).

Pore-cleansing strips   These low-tech at-home pore-cleansing strips can clear blackheads and open clogged pores. You apply the strip to your skin and quickly pull it off, ideally removing the plug of oil and the clog of dry skin cells. Mostly likely, you'll see tiny dots of debris adhering to the strip when you pull it away. Unfortunately, pore strips aren't a long-term acne fix, and they must be used in combination with a topical skin care regimen (brand names: *Biore, Pond's, Neutrogena*).

Prescription Treatments

The good news is that there are many new prescription topical treatments. These include new formulations with new vehicles that decrease irritation, improve efficacy, or, by combining two active ingredients, make the process more user-friendly. All of the principles described earlier apply here, too: the product must be applied on a consistent daily basis to your entire face, not just to acne spots, and any irritation or dryness (if not resolved with a non-comedogenic moisturizer) should be reported to your health care professional.

If you are not seeing results with your at-home skin care program, it is important to find a health care practitioner who will design a treatment program that takes into account the type and distribution of your acne.

The topical and oral prescription medication list below is abbreviated. Many times, picking an agent from one category and using it in conjunction with an agent from another category will provide the best result. Unfortunately, medicine is not an exact science and sometimes, if you have more resistant acne, it may take several months to get your condition under control. I will go into detail about special considerations in terms of skin color, pigmentation, and distribution in the case studies that follow.

Topical Treatments

RETINOIDS

Retinoids are the category in which the most advances have been made. The most recent research underlines the importance of incorporating a retinoid into your anti-acne regimen. Using a gentle cleanser, applying a moisturizer *before* you apply the retinoid, or using a retinoid on an every-other-day basis will reduce the chances of dryness and irritation. The following products are types of retinoids:

Tretinoin is available as a gel, a cream, a solution, or even in the form of slow-release micro-sponges. Tretinoin is unstable in sunlight, so apply it at night (brand names: *Retin-A*, *Retin-A Micro*, *Atralin*).

Tazarotene acts quickly to control acne. Available in a cream or a gel, tazarotene seems to be the most effective retinoid to shrink enlarged pores (brand name: *Tazorac*).

Adapalene is less irritating than others in this category. It is not affected by sunlight and can be used in combination with benzoyl peroxide. It is available as a cream, a gel, a solution, or wipes in different strengths (brand name: *Differin*).

TOPICAL ANTIBIOTICS AND BENZOYL PEROXIDES

Repairing skin-cell turnover is one of the keys to successful acne treatment. It's also important to control *P. acnes* bacteria. Reducing *P. acnes* can be done through the use of either benzoyl peroxide or a topical antibiotic. Topical antibiotics can have a side benefit of reducing inflammation and are often used for that purpose (brand names: *Metrogel*, *Evoclin*, *Clindagel*). The various products have different advantages:

Prescription-strength benzoyl peroxide   With the increased resistance of *P. acnes* to antibiotics, many physicians prefer to use benzoyl peroxide. Benzoyl peroxide is the knockout drug for *P. acnes*—and, unlike antibiotics, benzoyl peroxide doesn't allow the little bugs to develop a resistance to it. New formulations make it less drying. Be aware of the potential for bleaching any clothing, linens, or towels (brand names: *Brevoxyl*, *Triaz*, *Benziq*).

Azelaic acid   This antibacterial substance, which naturally occurs in grains, is an alternative to topical antibiotics or benzoyl peroxide for people with acne and pigmentation. Azelaic acid is best used in combination with other acne products and contains a natural bleaching agent that fights hyperpigmentation (brand names: *Finacea*, *Finevin*, *Azelex*).

Dapsone gel   This anti-inflammatory agent is very useful for acne patients with sensitive skin. It can be used in the morning or at night in combination with topical antibiotics or retinoids. However, if it is used with benzoyl peroxide, it discolors to a dark brown (brand name: *Aczone Gel*).

Combination products   Studies have shown that for most people, the most successful anti-acne approach combines a topical retinoid and a topical antibiotic, a topical retinoid and a topical benzoyl peroxide, or a topical antibiotic and a topical benzoyl peroxide. This can be done by mixing and matching from the products in this list or by choosing one of the new effective combination products now available (brand names: *Ziana, Epiduo, Acanya, BenzaClin*).

How to Get Your Best Results

You're the key to making sure that you get the most out of any topical treatment your doctor prescribes. Here are a few tips:

- Read and follow the instructions or prescription directions to the letter. If you have any questions, call your doctor. He or she would prefer that you call rather than be confused.
- Apply the medication to the entire face. If you spot-treat only, you are not preventing new lesions from appearing.
- Apply it every night.
- Use enough of the product to cover the entire face, avoiding sensitive areas like under the eyes or the corners of the mouth.
- Continue to apply topical treatments after your acne clears. Microcomedones continue to form below the surface, so treatment must be ongoing.
- Choose oil-free non-comedogenic makeup and grooming products.
- Apply topical acne medication before applying makeup.
- Give a medication time to work.
- Contact your physician about any irritation.

> **DR. AVA'S SKIN HEALER**
>
> When you apply spot treatments to an acne flare, use a clean cotton swab for each application to prevent the spread of bacteria.

Oral Medications

Sometimes acne just won't respond to a topical solution alone. That's why your doctor might recommend an oral medication, either alone or in combination with other acne treatments. Whereas a topical works from the outside in, oral medication addresses systemic issues and works from the inside out.

Whatever form of oral anti-acne therapy you're using, remember these do's and don'ts:

- Do take the recommended dose at the recommended time(s) every day. Maintaining a consistent level of medication in your system is important.
- Don't double your doses. More is not better, and it can be harmful.
- Do continue to take the medication until your doctor tells you that it's okay to stop. Treatment often fails when the patient stops taking the medication before it has done its work.
- Don't take any acne medication that has not been prescribed for you by your doctor. Taking a friend's medication or self-prescribing by buying online can be deadly.
- Do make sure that your doctor knows the truth about your health. Discuss any preexisting conditions and any other medications (over-the-counter, prescription, and even "natural" products or supplements) that you are taking.
- Don't hesitate to call your doctor about any side effects or to ask any questions you might have.

HORMONAL TREATMENTS

You may find it surprising that hormonal treatment of adult acne is on the top of my oral medication list. This is because it is the most appropriate way to treat the primary underlying cause of most adult acne: hormonal shifts. If you're a woman whose acne breakouts follow a characteristic pattern linked to your menstrual cycle, if you find that your acne flares up again as you near or go through menopause, or if the pattern of your acne includes your jawline, neck, chest, or back, you might be a candidate for hormonal anti-acne treatment. Because hormonal therapy affects your whole system, only your health care practitioner can determine if this is the best treatment.

Hormonal therapy is effective on its own, but in order to address the unwelcome companions of adult acne—wrinkles, brown spots, and textural changes—it is more effective to combine oral medication with topical acne medication. The following hormonal treatments are most commonly prescribed:

Oral contraceptives   These work by suppressing sebum-triggering androgen production in the ovaries, raising a protein (serum hormone binding globulin, or SHBG) in the blood that picks up excess circulating androgen, and reducing androgen production by the adrenal glands (brand names: *Estrostep*, *Ortho Tri-Cyclen*, *Yaz*).

Anti-androgens   Another approach is to block the androgen receptors on the sebaceous glands. Anti-androgens also can reduce the local conversion of androgen to the active dihydrotestosterone, reducing sebum production. They also can inhibit androgen synthesis by the ovaries and increase the level of a protein that binds androgens in the bloodstream (brand names: *Aldactone* generic name, *spironolactone*).

Hormone replacement therapy   Hormone replacement therapy (HRT) may suppress acne flares linked to the hormonal fluctuations of perimenopause and menopause. However, if your HRT includes testosterone, you may find that you are breaking out more than you ever did before. (See chapter 7 for more information about the skin challenges of midlife.)

ORAL ANTIBIOTICS

If you had moderate to severe acne as an adolescent, you may have been placed on long-term oral antibiotic therapy. Oral antibiotics control the *P. acnes* bacteria, but they carry a greater risk of systemic side effects than topical antibiotics do. In addition, the bacteria can become resistant to the medication over time.

Today, oral antibiotic therapy for acne is likely to be short-term and combined with topical treatments. You take the oral antibiotic just long enough to blast the bacteria—but not long enough for the bugs to develop resistance—and always with a comprehensive skin care program.

Not all oral antibiotics are suited to fight acne. The medication has to be able to penetrate the oil-clogged follicles, which penicillin, for example, can't do. Oral antibiotics for acne treatment generally come from two families, tetracyclines and macrolides:

Doxycycline   Tetracyclines are the most commonly prescribed oral antibiotic for acne therapy because they are effective and relatively cheap, but they have to be taken on an empty stomach four times a day. Doxycycline is a newer kind of tetracycline that can be taken once a day with meals (brands names: *Monodox*, *Adoxa*).

A low-dose formulation of doxycycline that is anti-inflammatory—originally developed to fight gum disease and now used in the treatment of rosacea—has been shown to be effective in combating inflammation from acne. The lower dosage means fewer potential side effects as well as avoidance of antimicrobial resistance (brand name: *Oracea*).

Minocycline   This is another new generation of tetracycline. It may penetrate more deeply into the sebaceous glands and work more quickly and effectively, with fewer side effects than either doxycycline or tetracycline. Minocycline should not be used long-term, however, because of its potential side effects, such as liver irritation. In addition, grayish-blue pigmentation may develop at the sites of previous inflammation, such as sun damage or acne scars (brand names: *Minocin*, *Solodyn*).

Azithromycin   This is a macrolide and is available under many brand names. It isn't as effective against *P. acnes* as the tetracyclines, and oral use makes it more likely that the bacteria will develop resistance. Nevertheless, it's an option for short-term oral antibiotic therapy if you can't take tetracyclines.

ACCUTANE (ISOTRETINOIN)

Accutane (its generic name is isotretinoin) is generally prescribed for patients with deep cysts or scarring or whose acne has been resistant to other treatment. It is derived from vitamin A and shrinks the sebaceous glands, restores cell turnover, and reduces inflammation. Its effects often outlast treatment, making it as close to a cure for acne as we have. However, it is not an appropriate choice for adult acne because of its potential side effects. Adult users can develop headaches, muscle aches, and thinning hair. In addition, it doesn't address the underlying cause of most adult acne, which is hormonal, so adult acne can return even after a course of Accutane.

Medical Procedures for Active Acne and Acne Scarring

Every month, new peels, lasers, light-based treatments, and radio-frequency treatments become available to treat acne and its ugly sidekick, scarring. I will describe the currently available (as of this printing) state-of-the-art technologies and procedures. I will also present some of my own case studies to address how these procedures can be tailored to address skin of color, different types of acne, and the presence or absence of acne scarring and pigmentary changes.

Chemical Peels

The most common medical procedure for acne is a series of light chemical peels. These can be AHAs, like glycolic acid, low-strength trichloroacetic acid, salicylic acid, or a combination of an AHA and retinoic acid. They are used to help clear blackheads, decrease papule formation, and promote faster cell turnover.

Comedo Extraction

A health care professional can use a sterile device that looks like a pen to remove noninflammatory comedones (whiteheads and blackheads). If a spa facial includes comedo extraction, be sure that the instruments are sterilized and the aesthetician is licensed.

Cortisone Injection

A dermatologist may speed the clearing of large acne blemishes by injecting them with low-dose cortisone. Consider this an emergency spot treatment, not a regular anti-acne regimen.

Intradermal Botulinum Toxin

The use of intradermal botulinum toxin type A (Botox) to reduce facial-pore size and excessive sebum production is a novel technique. According to a report in the *Journal of Drugs in Dermatology*, when Botox was injected into the skin for other purposes, patients reported improvement in skin quality and less shine to their skin. However, no current large-scale study has examined the use of Botox in the treatment of sebum production and pore size.

Photodynamic Therapy

One of the biggest breakthroughs in acne treatment came with the discovery that certain wavelengths of light can help to eradicate *P. acnes* without the side effects of systemic or topical antibiotics. One approach

---

Acne

A CASE STUDY

"She Looked Flawless"

Patient: Yun Suy, Asian, late thirties

I was a bit perplexed when Yun Suy first came to see me. She was absolutely stunning, with beautiful flawless skin. She started crying, "You have to help me! I'm breaking out all over!" What is going on, I thought? Nothing on her face. Where, then? She had breakouts on her chest and back—all stress-induced, a very common cause of adult acne.

Treatment Plan

Because I know that Asian skin is particularly sensitive to both laser and light-based treatments, I had to proceed cautiously in order to prevent discoloration or keloidal scarring. In addition, Yun had a sensitive stomach and couldn't tolerate medication to treat her acne. The alternative was to begin a series of photo-dynamic therapy (PDT) treatments to clear the acne and shrink the oil glands, as well as to eliminate bacteria.

In between her PDT sessions, she underwent a series of salicylic acid peels for her discoloration. I also prescribed a benzoyl peroxide wash for her to use once a day on her chest and back, along with a topical retinoid cream. Because the cream and the wash can be irritating, I suggested that she use a body lotion with soothing anti-inflammatory ingredients that included green tea, chamomile extract, and genistein. Her diet was already good, but I recommended that she add supplements, such as vitamin C, vitamin E, and niacin, to mute the inflammation associated with acne.

is to alternate between exposure to blue light, which kills *P. acnes*, and red light, which penetrates deeper into the blemish and reduces inflammation (brand names: *BLU U, Omnilux Red*).

We can also target and intensify the results of photodynamic therapy (PDT) by applying a photosensitizing substance to your skin before exposing it to light. This substance is absorbed by your sebaceous glands and activated by the light. It's important to stay out of the sun and away from bright artificial light for one to two days due to extreme photosensitivity (brand names: *Levulan, Metvix*).

Sessions are done at three-week intervals and, according to some reports, can give Accutane-like results. It is particularly effective on the back and the buttocks and is appropriate for people who want to avoid taking any oral medication but who have particularly resistant acne. You'll notice some redness and peeling, and you'll need to continue using topical agents.

Laser Acne Treatment

Lasers are used in acne treatment to destroy *P. acnes* bacteria, stimulate cell turnover, and shrink the sebaceous glands. You will need a series of treatments, combined with topical and perhaps oral therapies. Sometimes a fast-acting skin-numbing cream is applied prior to treatment to prevent discomfort. The possible side effects of lasers are some reddening or dryness for about twenty-four hours. In-office laser treatments for acne include the following:

Smoothbeam   This is a 1450-nanometer diode laser that treats active acne and acne scarring with bursts of laser light.

PDL   This is a pulse-dye laser that clears up redness from acne and rosacea (brand name: *Vbeam*).

Photopneumatic therapy   This is intense pulsed light combined with a vacuum that suctions debris from clogged pores. This therapy has shown favorable results with all forms of acne and, by reducing inflammation, lowers the incidence of the annoying brown spots that can occur after the acne goes away (brand name: *Isolaz*).

Acne

A Multiple Laser Approach

Patient: Jenna, Caucasian, late forties

My patient had a severe acne problem when she was a teenager that left her with some facial scarring—an unpleasant reminder of those earlier outbreaks. Now, because of stress and lifestyle changes, she had developed acne along her jawline, chin, and neck. Even though the location was different, it brought back bad memories of living with acne in her teenage years, and going through that drama again was extremely unappealing.

Treatment Plan

Jenna had new acne on top of old scars. So I decided to use a stepwise approach that included different types of lasers. I used the Vbeam, a vascular laser, to reduce the redness associated with her breakouts, in addition to the Smoothbeam laser, to treat her active acne, shrink the oil glands, and stimulate collagen synthesis to remodel her acne scars. Between these treatments, she received a deep-cleansing facial to clear her pores and a hydrating mask to add extra moisture to her skin—this was vital because her underlying skin type was dry.

After Jenna's active acne was clear, I used a nonablative resurfacing laser called the Fraxel Repair to further remodel the acne scars. At the end of her laser treatment series, I began her on a maintenance skin care program to enhance the results of those treatments, prevent a relapse of her acne, and continue the rejuvenation process. In addition, I suggested a change in her diet and fitness program.

She returned to me grateful, because for the first time in many years she could go to her son's piano recital wearing only blush instead of her usual pancake makeup.

Treating Discoloration and Scars

As we have learned, acne treatment doesn't end with controlling outbreaks. Because acne can cause scarring, discoloration, or both, it is especially important to have a real game plan to address the entire spectrum. The remembrances of blemishes past can often be even more troublesome and destructive to your self-image than the original lesions were. No matter what the topography of your skin, there are tools we can use to improve your appearance and confidence—often to a very significant degree.

Acne and even some laser acne treatments can cause persistent post-inflammatory hyperpigmentation (PIH). Although dark skin tones have an increased tendency to react to acne inflammation with discoloration, pigmentation changes can occur in light skin tones, as well.

Among the treatments your doctor can use to reduce discoloration are topical medications and peels that contain the following:

- Hydroquinone
- Azelaic acid
- Kojic acid
- Glycolic acid
- Salicylic acid

Your health care professional may also choose to use retinoids, either alone or in combination with any of the agents listed above. These active ingredients reduce blotchy pigmentation and restore natural skin-cell turnover. If they are drying or irritating, use in combination with a moisturizer. Unfortunately, any kind of laser therapy or deep dermabrasion can have unpredictable effects on skin of color, either darkening or bleaching the skin.

To reduce your risk of developing brown spots after acne (PIH), seek treatment at the first sign of breakouts. The faster you seek treatment, the less chance your skin will have of developing PIH in response to acne inflammation. Practicing strict sun protection is also important for the skin at all stages of acne treatment, because sun damage can trigger or worsen hyperpigmentation.

Acne causes scarring when inflamed lesions penetrate the deeper layers of the skin, doing damage to the collagen and elastin fibers that act as the skin's support structure. Only the most superficial scars can be completely eradicated. Otherwise, we aim for revision: altering the size, severity, and appearance of scarring to make a real difference.

Here are some steps you can take to ensure that you get the best results when seeking scar improvement:

- Keep your expectations realistic.
- Choose practitioners with experience. If you have darker skin tones, find a specialist who has experience with skin of color.

Skin Resurfacing

Resurfacing your skin to alleviate acne scarring is a paradoxical process. When we resurface the skin, we are actually creating a wound in order to prompt your skin's ability to remodel itself. By stripping off or other-

---

Acne
A CASE STUDY

Treating Skin of Color

Patient: Jasmine, African-American, mid-forties

Jasmine suddenly found herself breaking out with adult acne. She had never had a problem with acne before, even as a teenager. Though not severe, her breakouts were leaving behind a calling card: PIH, dark marks on her skin that were causing her almost as much stress as the acne itself.

Treatment Plan

Because skin of color contains a high melanin content, it is extremely susceptible to scarring, to developing light or dark spots, and to reacting negatively to a wider range of topical treatments. So I had to proceed with caution in treating Jasmine so as not to cause further damage.

First, I performed a light glycolic peel to address some of the general discoloration. This was followed by an Isolaz procedure, which uses photopneumatics to clear acne and reduce the dark marks. I prescribed a retinoid cream with hydroquinone to address both problems. Since retinol and hydroquinone can irritate the skin and lead to more discoloration, I also recommended that Jasmine add a moisturizer with anti-inflammatory ingredients to her regular skin care regime.

For the maintenance of healthy skin in the future, I suggested that Jasmine adjust her diet to include more anti-inflammatory foods, like fruits and dark green vegetables, and take supplements (such as vitamin A, vitamin E, selenium, and magnesium) to boost cell turnover and decrease inflammation.

wise damaging your skin down to the deeper levels, resurfacing damages the infrastructure of the skin and nudges the formation of new, healthier collagen and smoother epidermal cells.

The most common methods of skin resurfacing for the treatment of acne scars are the following:

Nonablative laser treatment   Nonablative lasers are used in photorejuvenation for their ability to plump the skin's underlying layers without doing damage to the surface. These lasers may be useful in remodeling some moderate acne scarring, but the effects are very subtle and may require multiple treatments. On the positive side, this treatment may offer a good alternative if you have darker skin tones or can't set aside the longer downtime that is required to recover from conventional laser resurfacing (brand names: *Smoothbeam*, *CoolTouch*, *Fraxel*, *re:store Dual*, *Palomar*, *Syneron*).

Chemical peels   Using chemicals to strip away the outer layers of the skin has become common in the skin care industry. Peels remove dead cells and brighten the appearance of the skin. Atrophic scars may look better after a chemical peel, but that's mostly due to the temporary swelling the chemicals cause. To resurface the skin down to the collagen level requires the use of highly corrosive acids, like those sometimes used to correct deep sun damage or wrinkles in fair-skinned people. Keep the following in mind:

- You'll need downtime so your skin can repair. Follow your doctor's instructions for keeping your skin clean and hydrated as you heal.
- Peels are most successful with fair skin, which won't show the lightening effects of the chemicals. If you have skin of color, consider other skin resurfacing options, or at least be sure that your doctor has discussed with you what you can realistically expect from peels.

Light peels are also effective in reducing scarring on the neck, chest, or back. Unlike the skin on your face, the skin in these other areas isn't thick enough to withstand harsher laser or dermabrasion resurfacing.

Fillers

Scar reduction and resurfacing may still leave you with an uneven facial landscape. If this occurs, or if your scars are fairly shallow and don't require more dramatic measures, we can even out the skin surface by injecting fillers below the scar. This is similar to the process of using fillers to smooth out wrinkles and lines in aging skin. Most injectable fillers are temporary. You may need to have more injections after your body absorbs the filler material. There is a permanent filler product that combines collagen with tiny plastic beads that will continue to provide support even after the collagen has been absorbed (brand name: *Artefill*).

A variety of natural and synthetic materials are used for filling in scars. These include the following:

Calcium hydroxylapatite Synthetically produced smooth microspheres are suspended in a sodium cellulose gel carrier for immediate one-to-one correction of deep acne scars. Over time, the gel is absorbed and fibroblasts appear. The process of neocollagenesis begins, during which the gradual growth of the patient's own collagen occurs. This helps to further fill in some of the depressions left behind by acne scarring. The results are soft and natural-looking and feel like the patient's own tissue (brand name: *Radiesse*).

Hyaluronic acid Also delivered in gel form, hyaluronic acid is a manufactured form of a substance that occurs naturally in the skin. It conforms well to the body and lasts longer than collagen injections. Hyaluronic acid shouldn't be used in very shallow scars, however, because light that passes through transparent skin layers will be refracted back by the filler, which will make the skin on the surface look dark blue—an effect that persists for months (brand names: *Juvederm, Perlane, Restylane*).

Poly-L-lactic acid This tissue stimulator (brand name: *Sculptra*) can be used to treat acne scarring. Sculptra is injected in a fanning fashion underneath an entire area, not specifically into a scar. It works slowly, requiring several injections sessions to build skin thickness and restore a smooth appearance that may last a year or more. If you receive these injections, be sure to follow your doctor's instructions for massaging the treatment area to prevent it from creating lumps. The formation of tiny bumps under the skin can occur, even if massage is performed.

Supplements That Heal Your Skin

You can get most of the daily recommended dosages of vitamins and minerals by eating a variety of healthy foods. Nevertheless, as Jeffrey Blumberg, a professor of nutrition at Tufts University, explains, "We can't rely on a few blockbuster foods to do the job. You can't eat nine servings of broccoli a day and expect it to do it all." Who would want to eat nine servings of anything a day?!

Instead, vitamin supplements can provide an antioxidant boost to help adult acne patients get faster results from their treatment plans. Supplements also nourish the skin and decrease inflammation and infection. People with healthy skin can use them for maintenance and prevention, especially if they are prone to outbreaks. However, not all supplements work for everyone. It is important to know what each supplement contains and in what amounts, and what effect it will have on your skin. In general, nutritional supplements for healing adult acne skin should contain some of the following:

Vitamin A   Encourages healthy skin, promotes wound healing, strengthens the immune system, and controls the development of the epithelial cell, which is a common component of the skin that lines all the mucosal membranes in the body.

Alpha-lipoic acid   Provides superior protection from free radical damage and inflammation. It is extremely valuable in treating acne because it helps to control the body's level of sugar and insulin. (A rapid rise in blood sugar can produce a burst of inflammation along with elevating the insulin level, which affects many other hormones in the endocrine system. This results in new acne lesions.)

DMAE   Dimethylaminoethanol is a naturally occurring nutrient found in high concentration in fish like salmon and sardines. In humans, it helps the brain to perform crucial functions and has also been shown to have anti-inflammatory properties.

Zinc   Found in more than two hundred enzymes that are important to our cellular health, zinc heals wounds, boosts energy and metabolism, and maintains collagen. Zinc is crucial to the proper functioning of the immune system and serves as an anti-inflammatory.

Essential fatty acids   Omega-3 and omega-6 are necessary for the performance of many biochemical processes in the body. Omega-3 fatty acids dramatically reduce the body's production of arachidonic acid, which is a major cause of inflammation. Omega-6 fatty acids are derived from linoleic acid, which has a widespread impact on the body because of its effect on membrane functions. Acne patients may have a low concentration of linoleic acid in the sebum, and the levels have been shown to decrease as the severity of the acne increases.

Vitamin B-complex   The interrelated B vitamins are known as coenzymes, which means that they help the enzymes to carry out their functions in the body. The B vitamins play an important role in energy production, nerve-signal transmission, and the synthesis of hormones.

- B_3 (niacin) has been used for years to treat inflammatory skin conditions, including acne.
- B_5 (pantothenic acid) is important for fat metabolism and may have an effect on sebum production in the skin.
- B_6 (pyridoxine) plays a role in the metabolism of steroid hormones.

Vitamins C and E   Both are antioxidants that mute the inflammation of acne. Vitamin E also hinders the aging of skin cells.

For overall good health, you should consider the following other supplements as well:

- **Tocotrienol**   Part of the vitamin E family, tocotrienol is excellent in fighting free radicals.
- **L-carnitine**   A substance related to vitamin B, L-carnitine prevents fatty buildup in the heart, the liver, and the skeletal muscles.
- **Calcium**   Excellent for bone health, calcium fights osteoporosis and hypertension.
- **Magnesium**   Necessary for more than three hundred biochemical

reactions in the body (such as muscle and nerve function, heart rhythm, and the immune system), magnesium also plays a role in hormone balance.

- **Chromium**   Chromiun enhances the action of insulin, a hormone critical to metabolism and the storage of carbohydrate, fat, and protein in the body.
- **Folic acid**   The synthetic form of folate, a B vitamin, folic acid produces and maintains new cells.
- **Selenium**   Selenium prevents cellular damage from free radicals and boosts the action of other antioxidants.

Dr. Wendy's Eating Well to Treat Adult Acne

We've all heard that junk food and chocolate cause acne, right? Actually, research tells us that this is not exactly the case. There is little evidence that chocolate or fatty fried foods cause acne, but we *do* know that a diet that promotes inflammation also promotes inflammatory conditions and responses in the body—including acne. Although we can't say that sugary or fried foods directly cause acne, it's nevertheless true that too much of these kinds of foods can increase inflammation and may displace other nutrients that *are* critical to the skin's health.

For example, filling up on sugary foods may lead to less consumption of fruits and vegetables. So it's a twofold proposition when it comes to acne treatment and the foods you eat for improving acne: you want to tip the scale in your favor by eating healthy, clear-skin-promoting foods *and* staying away from foods that decrease skin health or squeeze out essential nutrients. In other words, it's just as important to focus on what *to* eat to avoid or clear up acne as what *not* to eat.

Acne-Preventing and Clear-Skin-Promoting Food Tips: The What-to-Eat List

1. Stick to drinking water and green tea. Drink at least eight to ten cups a day—spread throughout the day, not gulped. Drink more if you're active.

2. Eat a fruit or a vegetable at *every* meal.

3. Have a vegetable-based soup or a garden salad every day.

4. Enjoy a handful of nuts per day (e.g., twenty-three almonds, fourteen walnuts, or forty-nine pistachios).

5. Use healthy oils exclusively: extra-virgin olive oil, grape seed oil, flaxseed oil, walnut oil, avocado oil. Eliminate corn oil, safflower oil, and sunflower oil.

6. Eat lean proteins to balance the glycemic response.

7. Consume omega-3 rich fish two or three times a week or take a daily fish oil supplement.

8. Eat mostly whole foods and very few processed foods.

Guidelines for an Anti-Acne Diet

- Eat more fruits and vegetables.
- Eat reasonable portions. Avoid too much food—both over the course of the day and at one time.
- Choose lean cuts of meat instead of those with more fat.
- Consume low-fat dairy, like fat-free or low-fat milk and yogurt, instead of whole-fat varieties.
- Prepare foods by grilling, baking, or steaming instead of frying.
- Season foods with anti-inflammatory flavorful herbs and spices instead of salt, sugar, and fat.
- Use herb- and spice-based healthy oil and citrus marinades instead of barbecue sauce (which is high in sugar).
- Drink plenty of water and green tea and avoid "liquid candy" (sugary beverages).

Acne-Fighting Nutrients

Getting adequate amounts of five key nutrients, preferably from fresh foods, is critical to fighting acne from within. Think of these fabulous five—let's call them ABCZ3 for short—as an oral prescription for clearer skin.

A = vitamin A (beta-carotene)

B = B vitamins

C = vitamin C

Z = zinc

3 = omega-3 fatty acids

A well-balanced, nutritious, skin-boosting diet offers all of these.

The Stress Factor: Are You a Stress Eater?

Chronic stress can be bad news for the skin. It contributes to acne flares by triggering inflammation and by motivating stress eating, which often involves poor nutritional choices. Here are some hints for making better food choices when you are feeling stressed out:

- Stock up on grab-and-go, finger-friendly snacks like blueberries, cherry or grape tomatoes, baby carrots, hummus, low-fat yogurt, and whole-grain crackers.
- Package snacks in advance in portion-controlled bags and containers to minimize overeating.
- Keep pro-inflammatory junk foods out of the house.
- Eat on a schedule.
- Drink a cup of water at the first sign of hunger—real or false.
- Have a cup of green tea for an antioxidant boost.
- Stay out of the kitchen when it's not mealtime or snack time.
- Take a five-minute walk along with ten deep breaths. This can break the connection between stress and eating and will ease your feelings of being out of control.
- Post a list of alternative activities—activities you can try *instead* of eating—on your refrigerator. This will intercept you when you're on autopilot, reaching for food when stress clouds your ability to think clearly.

Alisa's Fitness Tips

Have you ever noticed how much better your skin looks after a good night's sleep or when you've decided to walk or ride your bike instead of driving for a few days? Adult acne is a complex skin condition, but there are definitely some healthy habits that will start you on your way to a clearer complexion. On top of that list is exercise.

Exercise is so good for your skin because it combats stress, which is a major cause of adult acne. Cardiovascular exercise combats the secretion of corticoid steroids and has anti-inflammatory benefits that fight the look of stressed-out skin. It also boosts your immune system, which results in fewer breakouts. Undo the tension displayed on your face and regulate your stress hormones by starting your day with forty-five to sixty minutes on the treadmill or a brisk walk outside. Yoga and tai chi are also great ways to decrease stress and will help you to stay in the moment. So will any athletic activity that forces calm concentration and gives your mind and body a break from thinking stressful and destructive thoughts. As you exercise the stress out of your life, be sure to keep these tips in mind:

- **Don't overdo it!** We've all been in exercise classes with people who are intent on outshining the rest of us. Let them. You're working out to relieve stress, not to give yourself something else to stress about.
- **Pick fun activities.** If you don't like what you're doing, try something else. Take on something you've never done before. Yoga, hiking, a Zumba class? Our minds are programmed to pursue and accomplish goals. When we achieve those goals, we are rewarded with the chemical release of endorphins.
- **Add some resistance.** Resistance training with bands, machines, and free weights manages blood sugar, thereby reducing the need for insulin in the body. Insulin resistance—caused by unstable glucose levels—is linked to adult female acne and the intricate hormonal balances within the body. Resistance training three to four times a week will regulate blood sugar storage in your muscles and reduce insulin secretion.
- **Be intense.** Your immune system will fight off acne if you keep it strong. A great way to strengthen your immune system is to do some moderately intense aerobic exercise on a regular basis. A dedicated routine of brisk walking five or six days a week for a minimum of forty-five minutes a day decreases the risk of infection and boosts immunity the natural way.

- **Make sure you eat right.** Some great pre- and postworkout food combinations are eating lean proteins along with healthy carbohydrates in modest portions. Examples include oatmeal and egg whites or a small sweet potato and turkey breast.
- **Get plenty of sleep.** Exercise can lower your stress, but if you have trouble falling asleep, avoid exercising within four hours of going to bed,
- **Work on your posture.** Hold your head high, walk tall, and stand straight to elevate your spirit. These adjustments send positive messages to your brain—and to everyone around you.

Physical intimacy is a great form of exercise. Enough said!

Skin Care Regimens for Adult Acne

OILY SKIN

MORNING REGIMEN

Step	Directions
Cleanse	Wash with a cleanser that contains salicylic acid or glycolic acid.
Tone	If needed, gently wipe your face with an oil-controlling toner or apply serum.
Eyes	Gently dot a small amount of cream around the eyes. Choose products with ingredients that address your areas of concern. Vitamin K, retinol, caffeine, vitamin C, yarrow, horse chestnut, and gingko biloba address dark circles. Haloxyl, caffeine, vitamin C, cucumber extract, green tea, and aloe vera address puffiness. Hyaluronic acid, silica, soy proteins, acai berry, aloe vera, seaweed extracts, GABA, and argireline address wrinkles, firmness, and elasticity.
Prescription	Apply topical anti-acne medication as prescribed by your doctor.

Moisturize	Every day:
	
	    Apply a small amount of a light, oil-free, non-comedogenic moisturizer with antioxidants.
	
	If your prescription acne treatment has left your skin irritated or flaky:
	    Apply a light, oil-free moisturizer before applying your topical anti-acne medication.

If you have additional skin care needs:

Choose an oil-free moisturizer with ingredients designed to address your specific skin care issues. Salicylic acid, benzoyl peroxide, retinol (for evening use only), and azelaic acid address oil production and breakouts. Green tea, calendula, cucumber, aloe vera, chamomile, thyme, willow herb, perilla leaf extract, feverfew, red clove, evening primrose oil, zinc, mallow, red algae, silymarin, and ginger address inflammation and irritation. Hydroquinone, mulberry extract, niacinamide, arbutin (bearberry extract), licorice extract, kojic acid, and azelaic acid address brown spots. Retinol, vitamin C, alpha-lipoic acid, caffeine, copper peptide, ferulic acid, basil, grape seed extract, lutein, lycopene, pomegranate, green tea, coenzyme Q10 (ubiquinone), ginseng, genistein (soy isoflavone), and silymarin address wrinkles.

Protect	Apply an oil-free, non-comedogenic sunblock *every day*. *Note:* If your moisturizer contains a sunscreen of at least SPF 25 that blocks UVA and UVB rays, you don't need to add extra sunblock.

EVENING REGIMEN

Step	Directions
Cleanse	Wash with a cleanser that contains salicylic acid or glycolic acid.
Tone	If needed, gently wipe your face with toner or apply serum.
Eyes	Gently dot a small amount of cream around the eyes. Choose products with ingredients that address your areas of concern. Vitamin K, retinol, caffeine, vitamin C, yarrow, horse chestnut, and gingko biloba address dark circles. Haloxyl, caffeine, vitamin C, cucumber extract, green tea, and aloe vera address puffiness. Hyaluronic acid, silica, soy proteins, acai berry, aloe vera, seaweed extracts, GABA, and argireline address wrinkles, firmness, and elasticity.
Prescription	Apply topical anti-acne medication as prescribed by your doctor.
Moisturize	Every evening: Apply a small amount of a light, oil-free, non-comedogenic moisturizer with antioxidants. If your prescription acne treatment has left your skin irritated or flaky: Apply a light, oil-free moisturizer before applying topical anti-acne medication. If you have additional skin care needs: Choose an oil-free moisturizer with ingredients designed to address your specific skin care issues. Salicylic acid, benzoyl peroxide, retinol (for evening use only), and azelaic acid address oil production and breakouts. Green tea, calendula, cucumber, aloe vera, chamomile, thyme, willow herb, perilla leaf extract, feverfew, red clove, evening primrose oil, zinc, mallow, red algae, silymarin, and ginger address inflammation and irritation. Hydroquinone,

mulberry extract, niacinamide, arbutin (bearberry extract), licorice extract, kojic acid, and azelaic acid address brown spots. Retinol, vitamin C, alpha-lipoic acid, caffeine, copper peptide, ferulic acid, basil, grape seed extract, lutein, lycopene, pomegranate, green tea, coenzyme Q10 (ubiquinone), ginseng, genistein (soy isoflavone), and silymarin address wrinkles.

INGREDIENTS TO AVOID

Cocoa butter, coconut oil, peppermint oil, cinnamon oil, mineral oil, jojoba oil

AT-HOME TREATMENTS

You can purchase over-the-counter masks and exfoliates for oily skin, or you can make your own (see chapter 11).

Masks	You can apply a mask once or twice a week to reduce redness and inflammation from acne and to tighten the pores and temporarily reduce excessive oil production.
Exfoliation	As long as your skin is relatively calm, you can use a gentle exfoliating scrub once a week. If you are experiencing an acne flare-up or excessive oil production, do not use any kind of scrub.

IN-OFFICE PROCEDURES

Peel	Deep-cleansing facial	Laser treatment	Light therapy

COMBINATION SKIN

MORNING REGIMEN

Step	Directions
Cleanse	Wash with a gentle nonsoap cleanser that contains tea tree oil or aloe vera.
Tone	Gently wipe your face with a hydrating toner that contains rosewater and oatmeal. You can use glycolic acid pads or oil-control gel on the T-zone.
Eyes	Apply a small amount of cream around the eyes. Choose products with ingredients that address your areas of concern. Vitamin K, retinol, caffeine, vitamin C, yarrow, horse chestnut, and gingko biloba address dark circles. Haloxyl, caffeine, vitamin C, cucumber extract, green tea, and aloe vera address puffiness. Hyaluronic acid, silica, soy proteins, acai berry, aloe vera, seaweed extracts, GABA, and argireline address wrinkles, firmness, and elasticity.

Prescription	Apply topical anti-acne medication as prescribed by your doctor.

Moisturize	Every day:
	    Use an AHA hydrating lotion.
	If your prescription acne treatment has left your skin irritated or flaky:
	    Apply moisturizer before your topical medication.

Protect	Apply sunblock *every day*. *Note:* If your moisturizer contains a sunscreen of at least SPF 25 that blocks UVA and UVB rays, you don't need to add extra sunblock.

EVENING REGIMEN

Step	Directions
Cleanse	Wash your face with a cleanser that contains a low percentage of glycolic acid.
Tone	Use a hydrating toner all over the face. If needed, you can use glycolic acid pads on the T-zone.
Eyes	Apply a small amount of cream around the eyes. Choose products with ingredients that address your areas of concern. Vitamin K, retinol, caffeine, vitamin C, yarrow, horse chestnut, and gingko biloba address dark circles. Haloxyl, caffeine, vitamin C, cucumber extract, green tea, and aloe vera address puffiness. Hyaluronic acid, silica, soy proteins, acai berry, aloe vera, seaweed extracts, GABA, and argireline address wrinkles, firmness, and elasticity.
Prescription	Apply topical anti-acne medication as prescribed by your doctor.

Moisturize	Every evening:
	    Apply a light moisturizing lotion that contains antioxidants.
	
	If your prescription acne treatment has left your skin irritated or flaky:
	    Apply a moisturizer with anti-inflammatory ingredients before applying your topical acne medication.
	
	If you have additional skin care needs:
	    Choose a moisturizer with ingredients designed to address your specific skin care issues. Azelaic acid, salicylic acid, glycolic acid, retinol (for evening use only), tea tree oil, and zinc address oil production and T-zone breakouts. Hyaluronic acid, ceramides, olive oil, dexpanthenol (pro-vitamin B_5), evening primrose oil, borage seed oil, and colloidal oatmeal address extra skin hydration. Aloe vera, green tea, calendula, cucumber, thyme, chamomile, willow herb, perilla leaf extract, feverfew, red clove, evening primrose oil, and zinc address inflammation and irritation. Niacinamide, kojic acid, mulberry extract, vitamin C, pycnogenol (pine bark extract), strawberry begonia, and magnesium ascorbyl phosphate address brown spots. Retinol, caffeine, green tea extract, coen-

zyme Q10 (ubiquinone), carrot extract, rosemary, grape seed extract, genistein (soy), copper peptide, ferulic acid, lutein, rosemary, basil, ginkgo biloba, and vitamin C address wrinkles.

INGREDIENTS TO AVOID

Cocoa butter, coconut oil, peppermint oil, cinnamon oil, mineral oil, jojoba oil

AT-HOME TREATMENTS

You can purchase over-the-counter masks and exfoliates for combination skin, or you can make your own (see chapter 11).

Masks	Your skin will benefit from using a mask once or twice a week to deliver hydration and high concentrations of nutrients.
Exfoliation	Using a fine-textured scrub, you may exfoliate once a week to remove the top layer of dead skin cells. Don't exfoliate if you have very sensitive skin or if your acne medication causes irritation.

IN-OFFICE PROCEDURES

Peel	Microdermabrasion	Cleansing and hydrating facial treatment	Laser treatment

DRY SKIN

MORNING REGIMEN

Step	Directions
Cleanse	Wash with a gentle, soothing nonfoaming cleanser or use cold cream or facial cleansing oil.
Tone	Spritz your face with antioxidant spray and follow quickly with the application of a hydrating serum.
Eyes	Gently dot a small amount of cream around the eyes. Choose products with ingredients that address your areas of concern. Vitamin K, retinol, caffeine, vitamin C, yarrow, horse chestnut, and gingko biloba address dark circles. Haloxyl, caffeine, vitamin C, cucumber extract, green tea, and aloe vera address puffiness. Hyaluronic acid, silica, soy proteins, acai berry, aloe vera, seaweed extracts, GABA, and argireline address wrinkles, firmness, and elasticity.

Prescription	Apply topical anti-acne medication as prescribed by your doctor.
Moisturize	Apply moisturizer while your skin is still damp from the hydrating serum.
Protect	Apply sunblock every day. *Note:* If your moisturizer contains a sunscreen of at least SPF 25 that blocks UVA and UVB rays, you don't need to add extra sunblock.

EVENING REGIMEN

Step	Directions
Cleanse	Wash your face with a nonsoap cleanser that contains calendula, chamomile, or other soothing ingredients.
Tone	Apply facial water, hydrating toner, or serum.
Eyes	Apply a small amount of cream around the eyes. Choose products with ingredients that address your areas of concern. Vitamin K, retinol, caffeine, vitamin C, yarrow, horse chestnut, and gingko biloba address dark circles. Haloxyl, caffeine, vitamin C, cucumber extract, green tea, and aloe vera address puffiness. Hyaluronic acid, silica, soy proteins, acai berry, aloe vera, seaweed extracts, GABA, and argireline address wrinkles, firmness, and elasticity.
Prescription	Apply topical anti-acne medication as prescribed by your doctor.

Moisturize	Every evening:
	    While your skin is still damp, apply a moisturizer that contains moisture-locking ingredients like ceramides and peptides.
	
	If your prescription acne treatment has left your skin irritated or flaky:
	    Apply moisturizer before applying medication.
	
	If you have additional skin care needs:
	    Choose a moisturizer with ingredients designed to address your specific skin care issues. Hyaluronic serum, ceramides, glycerin, olive oil, dexpanthenol (provitamin B$_5$), and evening primrose oil address hydration. Aloe vera, green tea, calendula, cucumber, thyme, and chamomile address inflammation and irritation. Mulberry extract, arbutin, and pycnogenol (pine bark extract) address brown spots. Retinol, carrot extract, rosemary, grape seed extract, genistein (soy isoflavone), caffeine, copper peptide, and ferulic acid address wrinkles.

INGREDIENTS TO AVOID

Benzoyl peroxide, cocoa butter, coconut oil, peppermint oil, cinnamon oil

AT-HOME TREATMENTS

You can purchase over-the-counter masks and exfoliates for dry skin, or you can make your own (see chapter 11).

Masks	Masks can hydrate, reduce irritation, and soothe your skin. You can use a simple home-made mask or purchase one over-the-counter. Make sure the mask is specifically made for sensitive skin. If you have an acne or rosacea flare, talk to your doctor before using a mask on your face or your body.
Exfoliation	Only use very gentle facial exfoliants. Always make sure that the exfoliant contains no fragrance or chemicals. Homemade scrubs are a good option. If your skin is very sensitive, you can exfoliate with dry oatmeal (see the recipe in chapter 11). Do not use any peels or other microdermabrasion kits.

IN-OFFICE PROCEDURES

Cleansing and hydrating facial treatment   Laser treatment

9

Cancer Treatment

RENEWING YOUR SKIN

Sandra Bullock's beloved mother passed away after a long struggle with colorectal cancer. "My mother didn't lose her hair when she had chemo," the actress told me. "We have enough hair in our family to weave a rug or clothe an entire village. But her skin was extremely dry, and she felt like her nerve endings were on fire. Everything that touched her skin had to be extra soft, and she was constantly applying moisturizer."

I learned more about the importance of skin care during cancer treatment when Nancy Daly came to see me during her chemotherapy. Nancy had a very busy life. She was a wife and mother, ran a large children's charity, and was a board member of the Los Angeles County Museum of Art and the Los Angeles Opera. And she had no intention of letting a diagnosis of pancreatic cancer slow her down.

Nancy experienced a multitude of skin side effects from her cancer therapies. She taught me how important it is to give patients undergoing cancer treatment skin that not only looks good but feels good. Because of Nancy, I also began to realize that there is a large population who suffer from skin conditions induced by cancer treatment but who also have nowhere to turn with questions about skin care. What could they do to look good and feel better before, during, and after cancer treatment so that like Nancy they could still maintain their busy lives?

Cancer treatment isn't easy on the skin. How you take care of your skin as you go through treatment can impact not only your quality of life but also your emotional well-being. Cancer patients expect to lose their hair, have gastrointestinal issues such as nausea and vomiting, and experience fatigue. But they may be unaware, and therefore unprepared, for how cancer treatment will affect their skin. This can affect their progress and the success of their treatment, according to a landmark 2008 study.

Fortunately, no matter what those skin side effects are, there is plenty you can do to minimize the worst. You do not have to be a passive bystander. There are steps you can take to prepare your skin for treatment, and things you can do to make yourself more comfortable (or, at least, less uncomfortable) and to help your skin look better during treatment. There are skin-recovery steps you can take between chemotherapy courses. And there are numerous skin care maintenance and rejuvenation options available when you've completely finished your chemotherapy sessions.

Always remember the healing power of touch. You may feel as if you don't want your skin touched by anyone right now, but studies have shown the value of simple human contact. It connects us, it soothes us, and it definitely has healing properties.

Perhaps the most important thing you can do—and I say this over and over to my patients—is to take heart. Your mantra during this time is to remember that whatever is happening to your skin, no matter how dismaying: "It's only temporary." Every single side effect is treatable and negotiable. Although there's no way I can tell you that your skin will resemble the bloom of youth during this time—it won't—what I *can* say is that in the long run, with proper restorative care, your skin may very well look and feel even better than it did before you embarked on your cancer treatment.

So many of my patients have told me that guidelines and information about caring for their skin during this period were simply not available to them. They sought advice from fellow patients, because even their health care providers often lacked the information they sorely needed.

This chapter is a direct result of what I've learned from talking to other dermatologists and oncologists as well as treating patients who have undergone cancer therapies. It is designed to provide information on the myriad of potential side effects, preventive measures, and treatments for some of the skin-related problems you may experience. In this chapter you will learn:

- How some cancer treatments affect the skin
- How to care for your skin before, during, and after cancer treatment
- The most common skin side effects from cancer treatment
- How to heal your skin: The Dr. Ava Plan
- How to reclaim your skin's vitality after your diagnosis
- Nutrition and fitness tips
- Skin care regimens during and after cancer treatment

How Cancer Treatment May Affect Your Skin

Once you've been diagnosed, you and your oncology team will develop a treatment plan. Various forms of cancer treatment are available and are often used in combination. The decision may be based on the type and stage of cancer, its (and your) genetic profile, and other health considerations you may have. All cancer treatments affect the skin in some way. The reactions are frequently agent-specific and dosage-dependent. Almost everyone will experience some side effects, but the severity varies among individuals. Those side effects range from dry skin to body rashes.

Thankfully, most side effects clear up once you complete treatment. Because new drugs are being developed and new side effects are being identified, be sure to discuss all aspects of your treatment with your oncology team. Always describe any skin changes to your doctor or oncology support team. Be sure to listen to feedback from your own body as to whether a product or a procedure designed to soothe or heal you is actually performing its function.

Chemotherapy

This anti-cancer drug therapy delivers a cocktail of medicines that are toxic to cancer cells. Oncologists treat the cancer systemically, which means the drugs circulate throughout the body so as to be as thorough as possible and to ensure that no stray cancer cells survive to metastasize and replicate. Unfortunately, drugs strong enough to kill cancer cells can also be harsh on healthy tissue.

This means that every organ of the body is under assault, and your skin is no exception. In fact, because the skin cells are constantly turning over and remodeling, your skin may be subjected to more severe side effects than any other organ in your body. (See Table 9.1 for a more complete list of chemotherapy treatments and possible skin side effects.)

Chemotherapy affects the skin in four basic ways.

1. **Shutting down the sebaceous glands.** Chemotherapy drastically reduces sebaceous gland activity, drying up production of oil over the whole body. Dryness and dehydration to the point of pain can parch your skin, from your face all the way to your hands and feet, inside your mouth, your eyes, and even in your vagina.

2. **Exacerbating existing conditions.** During treatment, any skin conditions you already have (and may even have under control) can suddenly worsen in extreme ways, because chemotherapy literally damps down the immune system. Once the immune system is compromised, flare-ups of rosacea, acne, eczema, psoriasis, toe or foot fungal infections, photosensitivity, cold sores, genital herpes, and unusual allergic reactions are common.

3. **Triggering new skin conditions.** Certain anticancer drugs can cause skin side effects, such as an acneiform rash all over the body, painful nail beds, dry skin, mouth ulcers, and hand-foot syndrome (redness, swelling, and pain on the palms and the soles).

4. **Precipitating premature menopause.** Some chemotherapeutic agents can shut down the ovaries' production of estrogen, throwing the body into early menopause. For women over thirty-five, this is usually permanent. In pre-perimenopausal women (from puberty to early thirties), this estrogenic shutdown may be just for the

duration of the treatment. Low estrogen levels brought on by menopause can cause dryness, itchiness, flushing with hot flashes, rough skin texture, and the acceleration of the natural aging process.

Table 9.1

Some Common Systemic Chemotherapy Drugs and Their Skin Side Effects

Treatments/ Drug Types	Generic Drugs (Brand Names)	Adverse Skin Effects
Alkylating agents Nitrosureas	Mechlorethamine (Nitrogen Mustard) Cisplatin (Platinol) Cyclophosphamide (Cytoxan)	Redness and peeling Dark brown pigmentation in skin folds Hives
Antimetabolites	Cladribine (Leustatin) Gemcitabine (Gemzar) Hydroxyurea (Hydrea) Methotrexate (Amethopterin, Folex, Mexate, MTX) 5-fluorouracil (5-FU, Adrucil)	Swelling Itching Facial flushing Photosensitivity Nail malformation Tooth staining Flag sign (bands of hair discoloration)
Mitotic inhibitors Plant alkyloids	Docetaxel (Taxotere) Paciltaxel (Taxol) Vincristine (Oncovin)	Hand-foot syndrome (PPE) Itching Peeling of skin Swelling Nail abnormalities
Antitumor antibiotics	Bleomycin (Blenoxane) Doxorubicin (Adriamycin, Doxil)	Hand-foot syndrome (PPE) Nail separation Inflammation of actinic keratoses (sun damage) Skin darkening
Corticosteroid hormones	Prednisone	Bruising of the skin Fungal infections
Hormones Aromatase inhibitors	Trastuzumab (Herceptin) Rituximab (Rituxan) Anti-estrogen tamoxifen (Nolvadex)	Swelling in the mouth or on the lips Redness Rash Flushing Hot flashes Unusual hair growth

Targeted Treatments

Targeted treatments differ from chemotherapy because they target specific growth aspects or receptors of a particular tumor. Their use in cancer treatment is becoming more important and more widespread. In general, targeted treatments cause less severe side effects than chemotherapy (like nausea and hair loss), but they can adversely affect the skin.

In particular, a type of targeted treatment that blocks epidermal growth factor receptors (EGFR) often causes rashes. EGFRs are found in tumors, but they are also found in normal skin cells. By blocking or inhibiting the function of these receptors, EGFR inhibitors prevent cells from taking in messages ordering them to grow and divide. When this type of targeted treatment blocks the receptor of certain cancer cells, it slows the growth of these tumors or causes them to shrink. However, it also blocks receptors in the healthy skin, leading to skin changes. (See Table 9.2 for the most common targeted treatment drugs and their adverse skin effects.)

Immunotherapy

Immunotherapeutic drugs may jump-start your immune response to attack cancer cells or strengthen your overall immunity. They may also help your body tolerate higher doses of chemotherapy or other cancer treatments and moderate some of the adverse reactions.

Table 9.2
Some Targeted Treatments and Their Skin Side Effects

Treatments/ Drug Types	Generic Drugs (Brand Names)	Adverse Skin Effects
Epidermal growth factor receptors	Cetuximab (Erbitux)	Pimples
	Erlotinib (Tarceva)	Peeling, flaking
Tyrosine kinease inhibitors	Geftinib (Iressa)	Blisters on hands and fingers
Proteosome inhibitors	Imatinib (Gleevac)	Canker sores
Topoisomerase inhibitors		Infections around fingernails and toenails
		Hair texture changes
		Cracks in skin of hands, feet
		Pigmentation changes

Table 9.3
Cytokines and Their Skin Side Effects

Treatments/ Drug Types	Generic Drugs (Brand Names)	Adverse Skin Effects
Cytokines	IFN-α	Rash
	IL-2	Itching
	L-4	Flushing
	L-6	Canker sores
	TNF-α	Hair loss

Boosting your immune system has consequences. A revved-up immune system may leave you sensitive or allergic to otherwise benign substances. This may cause your skin to inflame, break out in rashes or hives, or become discolored. (See Table 9.3 for a list of commonly used cytokines, a category of cancer drugs that acts on the immune system, and their skin side effects.)

Radiation

Radiation to destroy cancer cells is sometimes known as radiation oncology, nuclear medicine, or X-ray therapy (XRT). You may receive radiation after surgery or chemotherapy to eliminate any stray cancer cells or to shrink a tumor before surgical removal. In this form of treatment, specific areas where tumors or cancer cells are present are bombarded with nuclear radiation that kills the cells.

Immediate skin side effects can be similar to severe sunburn: redness, itching, blistering, and peeling. Later the skin becomes very dry and flaky. The skin side effects of radiation may be intensified if you receive this therapy in combination with chemotherapy or other treatments. Radiated skin will eventually repair itself to some degree, but the skin in the treatment area may always be darker or lighter and drier than untreated skin. Skin exposed to radiation will also be permanently more sensitive to harmful UV rays, making rigorous lifelong sun protection a necessity.

Surgery

Surgery is the oldest known anticancer treatment, and it is still used for tumor removal when indicated. Depending on the type and stage of your cancer, surgery may be combined with chemotherapy, radiation, or other treatments. The possible skin side effects and complications of cancer surgery are similar to those associated with any surgery. However, scars may be slow to heal if chemotherapy or radiation compromises the integrity of the skin.

In women, surgery to treat cancers of the reproductive system may result in premature menopause, with attendant skin problems—dryness, wrinkling, thinning, fragility—resulting from estrogen depletion. And in some cases when the lymph nodes are removed as part of cancer surgery, you may develop lymphedema, a swelling under the skin caused by the buildup of excess lymphatic fluid. The swelling can be painful and may cause skin tearing that can lead to cellulitis, a serious systemic infection.

Preparing Your Skin for Cancer Treatment

In the same way that you prepare your body for a marathon by improving your fitness level, the best way to minimize the side effects of cancer treatment is to get your skin as fit as possible.

1. **Get a routine.** Whether or not you've maintained a regular skin care routine of cleansing, moisturizing, and protecting your skin from sun damage, you can start one now. The products that you use should be nourishing, fragrance-free, and nonirritating. Once your cancer treatment begins, you may need to adjust your skin care.

2. **Block the sun.** Because cancer treatment makes your skin extremely vulnerable to UV damage, now is the time to invest in a good sunscreen or sunblock, at least SPF 25, with broad-spectrum protection. Look for one that absorbs well and works with your skin type. Wear it every day, in every kind of weather. Buy a comfortable hat,

with a brim at least five inches deep all the way around, and a good pair of sunglasses with UV protective lenses.

3. **Refresh your makeup.** It's time to clean out your makeup kit and medicine cabinet. Cancer treatment will make your skin hypersensitive and increase the likelihood of contracting infections. Get rid of old makeup, dirty hairbrushes, used sponges, and skin care products past their shelf date. Be vigilant: make sure that everything that touches your skin during cancer treatment is clean, gentle, and free of irritants and potential allergens. To avoid a transfer of bacteria, you must be the only person who is using the products.

4. **See your dermatologist.** If you are seeing a dermatologist for an existing skin condition, such as adult acne or rosacea, let him or her know about your medical status. Your medications and treatments may have to be adjusted or suspended for the duration of your cancer treatment.

5. **Go to the dentist.** The mucous membranes that line your lips, the inside of your mouth, and your throat are skin cells, too, and therefore vulnerable to treatment-related side effects. To minimize these, make an appointment with your dentist to have a thorough cleaning, to repair cavities, and to adjust the fit of any dentures or other devices.

6. **Visit your hairstylist.** Hair loss can be one of the most upsetting side effects of cancer treatment. In interviews, cancer survivors and counselors both say that the moment a person doesn't recognize herself in the mirror because of physical changes caused by treatment can be one of the lowest points of the process. If you have long hair, consider getting it cut shorter. This will minimize the emotional impact of seeing your long hair fall out. Start shopping for wigs, even if you think you're going to shave your head or go bald. Experiment with wearing scarves or hats, and always choose natural materials like soft terry or cotton jersey because they are less irritating to the scalp than wearing something made out of a synthetic material.

7. **Prepare to pamper.** You deserve to be pampered now more than ever, so find a cozy spot in your home that you can devote to healing. Fill it with things you love—candles, music, favorite movies—anything that makes you feel better.

8. **Be tender to yourself.** Everyone reports some degree of skin tenderness. Buy soft cotton towels and bedding, sleepwear and undergarments, sweatshirts and sweatpants, socks and gloves. Launder them in gentle, fragrance-free products so that they are ready to enfold you in soothing warmth.

Skin Care during Cancer Treatment

Even the most mundane activities of your daily life carry risk, and if these are not adjusted to the special needs of your skin at this time, you can develop some unanticipated skin side effects. Before I talk specifically about how your skin might be affected during cancer treatment, I want to list some general skin-saving tips you should follow:

1. **Handle with care.** The skin is especially fragile at this time because it cannot regenerate itself in a normal way. Keep your soaps and cleansers free of drying and irritating detergents. Avoid any aggressive skin or hair treatments. If you continue to get manicures and pedicures, use your own sterilized instruments. Always clear any products and procedures (even a mani-pedi) with your treatment team first.

2. **Go fragrance-free.** Anything heavily scented that touches you now has the potential to irritate your skin. This includes the obvious, like perfume, but also can include toilet paper, facial tissue, scented laundry soap, dryer sheets, and fabric softener. Don't rely on the label "organic" or "natural" as an indicator that it will be good for your skin (brand names: *All Free N Clear, Trader Joe's Soap Free Laundry Detergent, Seventh Generation Natural Laundry Detergent*).

3. **Use a humidifier.** A humidifier, particularly in the bedroom while you sleep, is an excellent idea because it adds moisture to the skin and the hair. Be sure to choose one with cool or adjustable capabilities, a good filter, and a UV-antimicrobial feature so as not to spread airborne viruses, bacteria, and molds (brand names: *Vicks V3800 Cool Mist Tower Humidifier, Germ Guardian H-3000 Ultrasonic Humidifier*).

4. **Postpone aggressive exfoliation.** Many effective rejuvenation treatments, such as laser resurfacing and microdermabrasion, involve

deep exfoliation that removes the top layer of skin cells. During cancer treatment and immediately after, these procedures are too rough on fragile, sensitive skin. This also applies to at-home procedures.

5. **Wear gloves.** Hands are one of the most vulnerable parts of the body to experience dryness, cracking, and fissures because they're constantly placed under adverse conditions. For example, going from wet to dry too frequently can exacerbate dryness to the point of cracking and peeling. Wear clean, dry, long waterproof gloves—rubber or vinyl, if you're sensitive to latex—for all wet household chores and thin white cotton gloves for dry household chores. Do not wear gloves for long periods, and wash cotton gloves frequently. Applying moisturizer under the cotton gloves reduces friction from the glove and improves absorption of the moisturizer.

6. **Water and washing rules.** Since chemotherapy has already compromised your skin's structure, particular care is required when you wash or bathe. Avoid harsh products, hard scrubbing, pounding pressure, extreme temperatures, and long soaks. Shorten your showers and avoid saunas and steam rooms. Your skin is already parched, so it doesn't need to be parboiled in addition. If you use a washcloth, try flannel (it's softer than other materials). Use a freshly laundered one every time and don't share it with anyone. A used washcloth can be contaminated with fungus, yeast, or bacteria, increasing the risk of developing a skin infection. Soap sparingly and only in strategic areas—that is, underarms, groin, and feet—to avoid stripping the skin of much-needed oil. Unless you are actually dirty—for instance, if you've been gardening or hiking—you don't need to soap your body at all. Cleansing the face, however, is important to remove makeup or grime from the outdoors.

7. **Swimming rules.** Many people find swimming in a cool pool to be a refreshing break. If you choose to dip into a chlorinated pool, however, be sure to rinse off thoroughly afterward to remove potential irritants. Before going in, apply a thin film of Aquaphor Healing Ointment or another thick emollient on your hands and feet to prevent fissuring and cracking. Because of pollution concerns, it is better to stay out of lakes and oceans for the duration of

your chemotherapy. The last thing you need are water-borne viruses, bacteria, and fungi washing over your skin.

8. **Postbathing rules.** Vigorous rubbing with a rough towel can injure your skin. Use the towel just to absorb the wetness before you apply moisturizer. A moisturizer is most effective and absorbs most efficiently when your skin is slightly damp, so apply one immediately after bathing. Body oils are particularly good at soothing dry skin because they seal in moisture.

9. **See your doctor if you have an open sore.** Most anti-cancer drugs do not cause open sores. During chemotherapy, however, any minor scrapes, cuts, scratches, blisters, bites, and mishaps won't be able to heal as quickly. If you have a sore that hasn't healed after a few days, have it checked by your doctor to make sure it's not infected.

The Skin Side Effects of Cancer Treatment

How cancer treatment affects your skin (and hair and nails) will depend on your individual physiology and the drugs you're receiving. Side effects can occur right away or within several days, weeks, or even months of treatment. Always remember your mantra: Take heart! There are ways to cope with even the most severe skin complaints. I have listed the most common complaints alphabetically in a problem-solution format so that you can identify what these skin side effects are and the best way(s) to seek relief.

Acneiform Rash (Follicular Eruption)

When you are treated with chemotherapy drugs that target the EGFRs, you can develop a skin reaction known as an acneiform (or acnelike) rash. It can look and feel like severe teenage acne, but it can erupt everywhere. It's important to distinguish an acneiform rash from a new case or flare-up of adult acne—which can also occur as a side effect of cancer treatment—because the two are often treated differently.

Researchers have found that developing a rash while taking an EGFR inhibitor usually means that the treatment is working well. You can be premedicated with doxycycline before your course of treatment, and this often prevents the rash. An acneiform rash may appear about a week to ten days after starting treatment.

If you're not receiving targeted treatments and you develop a widespread rash, contact your doctor. It could be a sign of a serious allergic reaction to the chemotherapy drugs.

What to do: An acneiform rash is not like a flare-up of common acne. It is occurring on skin that is already dry and fragile from the cancer treatment. It can be tender, burning, and itching. If the rash is mild, you can try an over-the-counter low-strength salicylic acid or benzoyl peroxide preparation followed by a moisturizer that contains ceramides.

If the rash doesn't respond within a short period, ask your doctor about using a topical or an oral prescription antibiotic to relieve the symptoms and lessen the severity of the rash. Topical treatments include clindamycin, metronidazole, and a retinoid. Oral antibiotics include minocycline and doxycycline. Sometimes low-dose Accutane is required. These drugs may increase your skin's sensitivity to the sun, and it may take several weeks to clear the rash.

Burning Sensation

The sensation of feeling as though your nerves are on fire is extremely common among patients who are undergoing cancer therapies. It is not well understood, nor does it affect every person. This feeling tends to fluctuate, being worse at certain times of the day.

What to do: There is a prescription cream called Zonalon that may ease the sensation. Comfrey root extract, which comes in an oil, may also provide some relief. Using the softest-feeling garments (like flannel and pima cotton jersey) may help.

Cracked Lips

By their very nature, healthy mucosa—the type of epidermal cells that cover your lips—are rapidly dividing. This means that under normal conditions, your lips will repair themselves quickly after a cold sore or exposure to dry air. However, because most chemotherapy drugs target rapidly dividing cells, your lips may become painfully dry and chapped and may peel during treatment.

What to do: Take a slice of fresh, slightly chilled cucumber and apply it to your lips for a soothing, hydrating effect. You may also use pure aloe vera, pure coconut oil, or pure shea butter. (Avoid anything with added fragrances.) Keep your lips moist and resilient by using a lip balm. Avoid products that contain mint or citrus, which can irritate fragile tissue, or alcohol and glycerin, which are drying. Choose balms that contain ceramides (which replenish your skin's natural moisturizers), petrolatum, and antioxidants.

For daytime use, choose a lip balm that contains a sunscreen of at least 25 SPF. Buy several lip balms at once so you can keep them on hand— in multiple rooms at home, in your handbag, in your car, and in your desk at work—for frequent reapplication throughout the day.

If you wear lipstick, avoid the long-wearing varieties (they're very drying) or those that contain lip plumpers like capsaicin (pepper), which can irritate. Matte-finish lipsticks, especially in dark colors, tend to show peeling and cracks more prominently, so you may wish to go with light colors and shiny finishes. Lip gloss can serve as both color and balm.

Don't forget to hydrate your lips from within by drinking lots of water. If cracked lips become too painful, your doctor can prescribe a specialized moisturizer.

Discoloration

Cancer therapy–induced pigment changes appear in shades that vary with different inherited skin colors and ethnicities. Skin-color changes can range from yellow-green to greenish gray or slate gray. Nail-color changes may occur and can include unusual purple stripes. Some therapeutic agents may cause a darkening of the skin, especially in body folds and creases or in areas subject to pressure. Mucous membranes, including the lips, gums, lining of the eyelids, and even vaginal tissue, may darken or look yellowish.

Always have your doctor or dermatologist check any new or changing freckles or moles to eliminate the possibility of skin cancer, which may develop independently of treatment-related pigmentation. Most chemotherapy-related pigmentation changes generally resolve within a month or two after completing treatment.

What to do: While you are in treatment, there's not much you can do about pigmentation changes, other than disguising them with makeup if your skin is able to tolerate it. Many patients recommend mineral makeup because the microfine particles are gentler and less irritating to fragile skin than regular makeup is, but be sure to clear any makeup products with your oncology team. Do not use chemical skin lighteners or bleaches during cancer treatment, even if you used them before your diagnosis.

Dry Mouth

Both chemotherapy and radiation treatments can damage the salivary glands, causing dry mouth as a result of impaired saliva production. It can be temporary in the case of chemotherapy because the salivary glands will usually regenerate within a month or two at the end of the treatment. In addition, some painkillers, antibiotics, antinausea medications, antihistamines, and antidepressants can cause dry mouth. Being dehydrated or having an oral yeast infection (which is common when the immune system is impaired) can be contributing factors.

You know you have a dry mouth when you have thick mucuslike saliva and a sticky feeling. Your tongue may be painful or even feel as though it's burning. Cracks at the corners of your mouth (called *perlèche*) can appear and may become quite painful. Dry mouth causes difficulty eating because chewing, swallowing, and digesting food requires saliva. The decreased production of saliva can endanger the health of your teeth and gums because they need the constant rinsing action to take away bacteria and food particles.

What to do: See your dentist before your treatment begins for a thorough cleaning. During treatment, follow these tips to manage dry mouth:

- Stay hydrated. Drink small amounts of water throughout the day and every time you wake up at night. Keep a water bottle with you at all times. Try filtered or flavored water or eat sugar-free frozen pops if the chemotherapy drugs make water taste too metallic.

- Brush your teeth and your tongue after eating anything. Use a very soft toothbrush—a brush designed for young children is great—with fluoride toothpaste and gentle but effective strokes. Running the toothbrush under warm water before brushing will soften the bristles. Rinse your mouth with plain water after brushing. If you have mouth sores or if brushing causes bleeding (which can be a problem if your cancer treatment has lowered your blood count), you can use a moistened foam-tipped swab (but not a lemon glycerin mouth swab, because it's drying) to clear debris from your mouth. The gentlest setting on a water-jet cleaning device may also be used. Get back to brushing as soon as possible, however, because it's more effective for maintaining oral hygiene.

- Floss once a day using unwaxed dental floss. If some parts of your mouth are sore, avoid flossing there, but don't neglect the rest of your mouth.

- If you wear dentures, take extra care to keep them clean and free of food particles.

- Mix up your own soothing mouthwash with half a teaspoon of baking soda in four ounces of warm water. Swish this around in your mouth and spit it out. The baking soda will maintain the correct pH in your mouth, especially if you've experienced acid reflux or vomiting.

- Avoid dry or sticky foods.

- Many of my patients have found that the best thing they could do for their dry mouths was to eat watermelon or suck on frozen watermelon pops (no sugar added). Only watermelon works—nothing else will substitute.

- Ask your doctor about using an over-the-counter saliva substitute.

Dryness

Extreme dryness is the most frequent skin complaint among patients in cancer treatment. As my patient Jo explained, "Dehydration of the skin is beyond anything I could imagine. I just shriveled up." Dry skin is characterized by mild scaling, roughness, a feeling of tightness, and itching. Dehydration, extreme weather conditions, perfumed products, and allergies can contribute to dryness.

What to do: The best way to treat your dry skin is to use moisturizers regularly; they prevent water loss by layering an oily substance over the skin to keep water in or by attracting water to the outer skin layer from the inner skin layers. Ceramides are a particularly valuable ingredient; they replace a skin lipid that chemotherapy specifically diminishes. Take a short shower or bath, then pat your skin dry with a soft towel and apply a moisturizer immediately.

Olive oil, Lubriderm Bath Oil, or Neutrogena Body Oil can also be applied to your wet skin after you emerge from the bath or the shower. Use only mild, nonperfumed, nondeodorant soaps such as Dove, Basis, Aveeno, CeraVe, or Neutrogena. Wear cotton clothes next to the skin rather than wool, synthetic fibers, or rough clothing. Always wash clothing in a mild detergent and drink plenty of fluids, unless you are otherwise restricted. Avoid any products that contain perfume, such as bubble baths, soaps, and lotions.

Caution: If you are receiving radiation treatments, do *not* apply anything to the skin in the treatment area without clearing it with your medical team first. Many common ointments and moisturizers, while nonirritating, may interfere with the ability of the radiation to penetrate the skin and do its work.

Eye Irritation

Dry, burning eyes are a common side effect of all forms of chemotherapy. The same oil glands present in your mucous membranes in your mouth and on your skin exist in the skin around your eyes. When their oil production is diminished by the effects of chemotherapy, the tear film dries, causing dry eyes that burn and sting. One of my patients told me, "At night my eyes felt like burning embers."

What to do: Artificial teardrops can be used. If they don't provide relief, see your physician for prescription eye drops that contain clindamycin, tetracycline, or the brand Restasis.

Cancer Treatment Skin Care
A CASE STUDY

"A Wounded Animal"

Patient: Janet, Caucasian, sixty

Janet was a two-time breast cancer survivor who had just finished several months of aggressive chemotherapy when she came to my office for a consultation. Now that she had beaten the disease again, Janet was happy to be alive but was very unhappy with the toll it had taken on her appearance. Her skin was extremely dry, her cheeks were sunken, and her hair, which was growing back, had a brittle quality.

Janet thought that she looked like a "wounded animal." She told me about the time she'd gone to the grocery store to buy broccoli and paper towels. "Just those two little things," she said. "As I'm checking out, they ask me if I want help to my car. I thought, 'Oh, my God, do I look that bad?'" Then she saw her reflection in the store window. "I *do* look that bad!"

Janet wanted to know what we could do to address some of the skin-related damage caused by her cancer treatment so that she could show everyone how great she was feeling, inside and out. As she eloquently explained, "I want the joy that is in my heart to be reflected on my face."

Treatment Plan

Since chemotherapy had dried out Janet's skin, we began with a series of hydrating facials. Her scalp and her hair were also very dry, so she had a massaging oil treatment to nourish the scalp and add moisture to her hair regrowth. I used several different types of lasers to even out her skin tone and stimulate collagen. I also injected hyaluronic acid filler to add facial volume.

Prior to her cancer treatment, Janet had not been following a regular skin care regimen, so we developed one that included easy-to-follow steps for cleansing, moisturizing, and protecting every morning and evening. The regimen included products that would hydrate her skin with natural oils, rejuvenate it with antioxidants, and protect it from the sun. When Janet saw the results of adhering to a regular skin care plan, she became a big believer.

"I carried that regimen with me everywhere I went so I could always remember what I needed to do to take care of my skin," she later told me. Even when her home was evacuated because of fires in the area, "I had that plan in my pocket! I was not leaving *that* behind."

Janet came to my office a few weeks ago, and she truly is transformed. Her skin is healthy, her hair shines, and everything about her appearance now reflects a woman who is happy to be alive. "I never imagined I could look so fabulous," she said.

Hair Changes

It is a common misconception that every cancer treatment will result in hair loss. With today's targeted therapies, it's not as common as it once was. Many anticancer medications don't cause hair changes at all or have only mild effects. Changes to your hair may seem drastic, but they are temporary. Hair follicles are resilient and will begin regenerating soon after your treatment is completed—or even before. When the hair regrows, it may have a different texture, color, or shape.

HAIR LOSS (ALOPECIA)

If you are receiving anticancer drugs that are likely to cause hair loss, it may be partial or complete. You may lose not only the hair on your head but also your eyebrows and eyelashes, underarm hair, and pubic hair. Other body hair is usually finer and grows more slowly, so it won't necessarily be affected.

What to do: Plan ahead. Assume that it's going to happen, and you won't be as thrown by it.

You have many choices with cancer-related hair loss: you can skip cosmetic cover-ups or choose from a number of wig, cap, or scarf options. Your oncology team, other patients, and members of support groups like the American Cancer Society's "Look Good, Feel Better" program or The Wellness Community can be helpful in discussing your options.

Keep in mind, you will need to take special care of your scalp. The skin on your head, neck, and forehead will suffer from the same dryness, propensity to irritation, and increased vulnerability to sun damage as the rest of your skin during cancer treatment. In fact, it may be quite tender.

Here are some tips for dealing with hair loss:

- My patients recommend using witch hazel or a gentle baby shampoo to cleanse the scalp. Massaging the scalp gently with the fingertips can be soothing.
- Don't wear a wig or any other hair covering for too long a period in hot weather. Sweat can build up on your scalp and become very irritating.

- There are many different options for wigs: real hair, synthetics, different hair colors. You can be a redhead or a blonde! The most important aspect is the fabric of the skullcap (brand name: *Wonderlox Hair Bands*).
- Many of my patients like to keep their heads covered at night or in cool weather to prevent body heat from escaping. There are many styles of soft, stretchy cotton sleep caps available. These can also be worn to prevent irritation under scarves, caps, and hairpieces.
- Choose soft, natural, and breathable fabrics like cotton jersey for anything you wear on your head.
- Makeup can camouflage the absence of eyebrows or eyelashes. Never glue on false eyelashes. After your cancer treatment is over, you can talk to your doctor about using Latisse or other lash-promoting products.
- While your hair is growing back, avoid dyes, blow dryers, processing, and other chemical or heat treatments.

THINNING AND BREAKAGE

This can be the first sign of total hair loss, but it may also occur as part of a milder skin-related reaction to cancer treatment. Chemotherapy can make hair more brittle and fragile.

What to do: Treat thinning and brittle hair as gently as possible. Use mild, detergent-free shampoos and detangling rinses—in general, the products designed for babies are great. Talk with your doctor about whether you can take a supplement. Hair care products will not help.

COLOR CHANGES

Your hair color may darken or look dull during treatment because the hair shaft absorbs metals from some chemotherapy drugs. Targeted treatments, which don't generally cause hair loss, may result in hair color changes. This includes an effect known as a *flag sign*, in which the hair develops a light-and-dark-striped pattern. When your hair grows back in, it may be a different color or prematurely gray. These color changes usually aren't permanent, although you may stay gray if you are now in menopause because of the cancer treatment.

What to do: Don't think about coloring your hair while you are undergoing cancer treatment. Even gentle herbal hair colorings may be too much for fragile hair to take.

TEXTURE CHANGES

The texture of your hair may change, either during or after treatment. It may go from fine to coarse, from curly to straight, or vice versa.

What to do: You can't do much to combat hair texture changes that occur during treatment, other than cutting your hair or wearing a scarf or a cap. Keep your hair clean and moisturize both your hair and your scalp. Olive oil makes a good inexpensive moisturizing treatment.

UNUSUAL GROWTH

This side effect is much rarer than hair loss, but it can occur when targeted treatments incorporate hormones or steroids or cause premature menopause. You can experience an excessive growth of facial hair or eyelashes as well as a lengthening or darkening of body or facial hair.

What to do: Talk with your oncologist about ways to remove or camouflage excessive hair growth. If your eyelashes grow so long that they make it hard for you to see or wear glasses, have an aesthetician trim them; don't do it yourself.

Hand-Foot Syndrome

Also known as palmar-plantar erythrodysesthesia (PPE), hand-foot syndrome is characterized by dryness, redness, and irritation on the hands and the feet that is so extreme that they actually begin to crack and peel. It can be so uncomfortable that your extremities may burn, tingle, or feel numb, making walking and driving impossible.

To prevent PPE from happening, your oncologist may try cooling your hands and your feet while you're receiving chemotherapy by placing them in cold water or on ice packs. Other options include using the sleeves designed to quickly chill wine bottles as hand or foot wraps and wearing a special thermal glove (called the Elasto-Gel glove) that contains glycerin.

What to do: Always notify your oncology team at the first signs of tingling and redness in your hands and your feet. Your doctor may recommend or prescribe topical treatments that can soothe the irritation and keep the reaction under control. Other strategies for dealing with hand-foot syndrome are as follows:

- Moisturize your hands and feet with soothing, alcohol-free salves or balms.
- If the skin on your hands and your feet becomes very dry and scaly, you can use a gentle nighttime exfoliation to remove the buildup of dead skin cells. First cleanse the area with a detergent-free body wash and a flannel washcloth. Then mix a dollop of cream that contains AHAs, urea, or ceramides with a dollop of a petrolatum-based salve like Vanicream. Slather this mixture on your hands and feet before slipping them into cotton gloves and socks.
- If you develop a related rash under your arms or in your groin area, you may use cornstarch (not talcum) powder to soothe itching and control sweating. Avoid shaving or other hair removal in these areas while you are under treatment.
- Don't pull or tear hangnails; clip them carefully with sterilized clippers. Put away your sandals and wear closed shoes and socks by day. In the house, wear closed-toe slippers with your socks. Your socks should be cotton. Synthetic fibers can cause perspiration that can irritate unless they are designed to wick away moisture.
- Avoid any extra pressure or friction on your feet. Gel inserts may make walking easier. Look for Dr. Scholl's Massaging Gel Insoles or TheraPedic Cooling Insoles.

Itching

Itching often accompanies dry skin and is a side effect of many anti-cancer drugs. Itching may also indicate an allergic reaction, either to a treatment agent or to a common substance you wouldn't ordinarily react to with sensitivity. Some people treat itchiness with a hot bath and rubbing alcohol, which is the exact opposite of what you should do because it will dry out your skin even more and may even burn it.

What to do: Moisturize itchiness rather than scratching it. Colloidal oatmeal products in the form of baths or lotions can relieve dry-skin itching. You can make your own soothing bath by dissolving bath oil or olive oil and a cup of regular (not instant) oatmeal in a tub of luke-warm water and taking a brief soak. Cool compresses may provide some relief. For severe itching, talk to your doctor about using an over-the-counter or prescription antihistamine—but keep the moisturizing routine going.

Mouth Ulcers

Chronic ulcerations or sores inside the mouth that look like canker sores are another very common side effect of chemotherapy. Beyond uncomfortable, they can be so painful that they make eating difficult.

What to do: You may be able to prevent or lessen the severity of mouth ulcers by sipping ice water, holding ice chips in your mouth, or sucking on frozen pops during chemotherapy treatment. A prescription oral rinse such as Peridex or PerioGard is often effective in preventing these ulcers. If you do experience recurrent mouth ulcers, you should first have them cultured by your doctor to make sure that you don't have a bacterial or yeast infection, or a reactivation of the herpes simplex virus (which manifests as cold sores or fever blisters). If mouth sores cause intense pain or interfere with your ability to nourish and hydrate yourself, you may need narcotic lollipops or a specially compounded mouthwash that contains painkillers, antibiotics, and antacids.

For treatment of chemotherapy-related mouth sores, follow the tips for managing dry mouth and also do the following:

- Rinse your mouth with water frequently.
- Do not smoke or drink alcohol.
- Avoid spicy, salty, or acidic foods.
- Drink through a straw and use a small nonmetallic teaspoon to eat.
- Try over-the-counter canker medications such as Anbesol or Orajel.
- Puncture a vitamin E capsule (400 IU) and squeeze the oil onto a swab. Gently place swab on open areas.

Nail Changes

Changes to your nails will depend on the treatment you receive. They are usually temporary, although the nails may take longer to repair themselves than the hair and other skin cells. Nail toxicity can occur weeks or months after you've begun a targeted treatment, and it often persists for weeks or months after stopping the drug. These treatments tend to affect the toenails and the thumbnails more than the fingernails. The nail changes you might see include the following:

- General dryness of the cuticles and fragility, peeling, and crumbling of the nails
- Separation of the nail plate from the nail bed
- Pale or dark streaks in the nail plate, called hyper- or hypopigmentation
- Malformation of the nails, including curving and cupping
- Paronychia, an inflammation around the nail bed that can be quite painful

What to do: Nail changes often disappear when the damaged nail is replaced by the growth of a new nail. Good nail care during your treatment can help you to avoid or diminish the severity of the side effects.

- Moisturize the nails and the cuticles daily with a nonirritating balm, such as petroleum jelly. You can also use lip balm to soften the cuticles.
- Don't bite, pick, or peel your nails, chew your cuticles, or rip off hangnails.
- Keep your nails trimmed short and gently filed; be sure to use clean implements.
- Do not trim or push back your cuticles. The seal they provide around the nail plate prevents infection.
- Do not wear artificial nails or extensions, especially acrylics.
- If your nails begin to separate or show signs of breakage, try to keep them in place as long as possible. Even when loosened or shortened, they provide protection for the nail bed.
- Nail polish can be used to harden nails and prevent nail breakage. If your doctor permits using polish, choose those one that is free

of irritating formaldehyde, toluene, and DBP (phthalates). Using clear or light shades will allow your oncology team to better monitor any changes to your nail bed (brand names: *Suncoat*, *Revlon*, *Adoree*, *Zoya*).

- Avoid professional manicures during treatment unless your oncologist approves. If so, choose a clean, licensed, well-maintained facility and a nail technician who is familiar with cancer treatment–related nail issues. Bring your own polishes, removers, and clean nail implements. Don't allow the manicurist to cut your cuticles or remove calluses. Don't do spa pedicures. Your system may pick up bacteria from a shared whirlpool.

- Inform your oncology team if you see any signs of nail infection, such as swelling or redness around the nails, blistering, or crumbling.

- Inflammation can be treated in a variety of ways by your oncology team, such as by the use of a topical antibiotic, an antifungal, or a cortisone cream. Wrapping the treated area with a bandage or clear plastic wrap (such as Saran Wrap) will help the ointment to penetrate the area. Some also find it helpful to apply a liquid bandage to the area at the first sign of any cracking skin.

Peeling and Blistering

Peeling and flaking of the skin (desquamation) is often associated with radiation treatment and the dryness caused by chemotherapeutic drugs. Blistering is a more serious reaction of the skin to drug toxins. Blisters may appear as raised, fluid-filled bubbles on the skin or the mucous membranes and may ooze fluid. With radiation therapy, you may get a so-called *wet reaction*—blistering, oozing, and peeling—in treated areas where the skin is very thin or where there are folds and creases, such as under your arms.

What to do: Have your oncology team check any peeling, flaking, or blistering to rule out serious conditions. For mild flaking and peeling of dry skin layers, you may get some relief from very gentle exfoliation by using a detergent-free body wash and a soft washcloth moistened in lukewarm water. Do not peel your skin or pop blisters.

Preexisting Skin Conditions

Because you are under an enormous amount of stress and your immune system is compromised, cancer treatment can exacerbate a preexisting skin condition. You might also develop a new skin condition for the first time.

ROSACEA

Rosacea is characterized by redness, inflammation, and broken blood vessels, or telangiectases. Rosacea most commonly occurs in people with very fair skin who flush easily. It worsens with age and can occur anywhere on the face, but it is most prevalent across the nose and the cheeks. When chemotherapy is involved, rosacea that hasn't flared for years may suddenly announce itself with deep cysts and dense redness.

What to do: See your health care provider immediately to get your medication adjusted. Chemotherapy-triggered rosacea is not only painful and unsightly, its lesions can leave permanent scars. Avoid as much as possible anything that makes you flush: extremes in temperature, alcohol, spicy foods, exertion, sun exposure, and stress.

OTHER SKIN OUTBREAKS

Other conditions that might be triggered or made worse by cancer treatment include the following:

- Herpes viral eruptions of all types. Once contracted, herpes viruses remain dormant in your system until triggered by stress or immune deficiency. Cancer and cancer treatment may trigger flare-ups of cold sores, fever blisters, genital herpes, or shingles.
- Flare-ups of genital warts, caused by the human papilloma virus, are extremely common in patients who are receiving cancer treatment.
- Psoriasis, eczema, and seborrhea may be triggered by cancer treatment.

What to do: Let your cancer treatment team know if you have a history of any of these chronic skin issues. An oncologist can work with your general physician or your dermatologist to tailor a plan for controlling the symptoms. Always tell your oncologist if you develop any new or unusual skin symptoms.

Rashes

Rashes and rashlike eruptions are a common side effect of many drug treatments, including chemotherapy. Treatment-related rashes can range from mild to severe and can be localized or widespread. They may be only a simple cosmetic nuisance or can be accompanied by itching, tenderness, irritation, flushing, blistering, or skin peeling.

Side-effect rashes are linked to the type of cancer drugs you receive, the dosage, and your unique systemic and skin conditions. Different drugs cause different kinds of rashes. The word *rash* is actually a general term for skin reactions. Here are some specific terms that describe what the rash may look like:

- **Erythematous:** characterized by generalized skin redness
- **Macular:** small, distinct, red flat areas
- **Papular:** small raised lesions

A maculopapular rash is the most common type of drug-induced skin reaction. This rash is usually bright red in color, and the skin may feel hot, burning, or itchy. It can occur with almost any drug at any time up to three weeks after the drug has been given, but it is most common in the first ten days.

Other rashes may include the following:

Hives   These are raised itchy blotches that may be pale in the center and red around the outside.

Contact dermatitis   This is an allergic rash triggered by coming into contact with substances that cause a hypersensitivity reaction. Because cancer treatment affects the immune system and strips the skin of its protective layer, anyone who is undergoing treatment can develop new allergies to just about anything.

Purpura   This is a condition characterized by bleeding under the skin or in the mucous membranes, resulting in purplish spots or patches. The main cause of this reaction is a very low blood platelet count. See your doctor immediately.

What to do: Always have your treatment team examine any new or worsening rash to rule out drug allergies and other serious skin conditions. For relief of mild to moderate symptoms, follow the tips for dealing with dryness and itching.

Yeast Infections

Yeast infections are common in people undergoing cancer treatment because of their suppressed immune system. The two most common types are:

THRUSH

Thrush appears as whitish, velvety lesions in the mouth and on the tongue. Underneath the white material is red tissue that may bleed easily. The lesions can slowly increase in number and size.

What to do: Your doctor can prescribe an antifungal mouthwash (nystatin) or lozenges (clotrimazole) to suck on. If your mouth is especially dry or if you have other mouth ulcers, you can freeze the nystatin liquid in an ice tray to make a soothing frozen pop. Keeping your mouth clean and using a baking soda rinse to maintain the appropriate pH balance may ward off oral thrush.

VAGINITIS

Vaginal yeast infections can also occur. You might notice itching, burning, and redness of the vaginal tissues or a thick white vaginal discharge.

What to do: If you develop a vaginal yeast infection, your doctor can prescribe oral medications or direct your use of over-the-counter treatments.

Healing Your Skin: The Dr. Ava Plan

Here is what my patients really want to know: "How do I take care of my skin when it is under assault not only from the natural aging process, cumulative sun damage, and abrupt hormonal physiological shifts but also from changes brought on by cancer treatment?"

Maintaining a regular daily skin care regimen is critically important,

Cancer Treatment Skin Care

A CASE STUDY

"I Have a Problem"

Patient: Patricia, Caucasian, mid-forties

When Patricia came to see me, she was feeling frustrated. She had been diagnosed with Stage II breast cancer and was treated with a lumpectomy, chemotherapy, and radiation. She had done a lot of reading before chemotherapy began and knew what to expect in terms of nausea, her hair falling out, and so on—but no one ever explained how her skin would be affected.

"In fact, no one said anything about skin symptoms occurring at all," she lamented. "The first thing I noticed was a discoloration of my skin and redness. With subsequent treatments, my skin felt rougher, thicker, and rubbery. I had no idea if these changes were going to be permanent."

Treatment Plan

Patricia experienced some of the most common changes that are seen with breast cancer therapy. I began by reassuring her that all of the skin changes could be improved with topical treatments and that none of them would be permanent. I then designed a skin care plan that included the use of antioxidants, a ceramide-containing moisturizer, and a nondetergent chemical-free cleanser. She also began increasing her intake of superskin foods—fruits and vegetables—and supplements.

not only for your own sense of well-being but also for your health. Caring for your skin will keep it stronger and better able to withstand the assaults of your cancer treatment. Daily all-over skin care will also help you stay aware of any allergic reactions or irritations that can lead to infection. The goal is to keep your skin as healthy as possible so that you can continue with your treatment.

Here are five important rules that apply to your skin care:

1. Whatever products you choose, they must be like a good spouse (or boyfriend or girlfriend): kind and gentle. Don't use anything harsh or drying. This is not the time to shrink your pores or do

any type of aggressive at-home rejuvenation. Looking ten years younger will have to wait until you are through your treatments, but fear not, it can still happen even after chemotherapy.

2. Your skin care program must be hypoallergenic, fragrance-free, and free of common irritants such as detergents. Check for preservatives like parabens. Although preservatives are necessary to prevent contamination, some may now be the source of allergic reactions in your very sensitive skin. To avoid contact with any kind of chemicals, make your own skin care products using the homemade recipes in chapter 11.

3. Keep moisturizing. Your skin's need for extra moisture during cancer treatment is intense. Applying moisturizer or soothing balm throughout the day can provide relief from dryness, itchiness, and burning. My skin care program is applicable to the majority of patients; the only exceptions are those who are experiencing a specific rash, such as the acneiform eruptions that accompany certain targeted therapies.

4. Clear your use of all products and ingredients, even over-the-counter skin care solutions and homemade masks, with your oncology team. This is particularly important if you are receiving radiation because many skin care products contain ingredients that block radiation and would therefore interfere with the success of the treatment.

5. Keep things simple. Undergoing cancer treatment is exhausting on every level. Regular skin care is important, but if you make things too complicated, you might be tempted to skip it on days when treatment leaves you fatigued. It might be easier to write your skin care plan on a piece of paper for those times when it's too hard to concentrate on anything.

A note on product selection: Some patients prefer to stick with a single manufacturer for their skin care products. Others like to mix and match. Whatever suits you and makes you feel best is fine with me. In the basic skin care regimen that follows, I've singled out products that my patients like and that generally meet the requirement for gentleness during cancer treatment.

Phase 1: Cleanse

Remember that the key is to be gentle when you cleanse your skin. That applies to the temperature of the water, to the product you use, and even to your washcloth. Always cleanse with tepid water, never hot. Never scrub or rub vigorously. You do not want to tear fragile tissue or dehydrate any part of your skin. Avoid loofahs or anything with a rough texture. Use only an unscented nondetergent cleanser.

Over-the-counter facial cleanser suggestions include: Cetaphil Facial Cleanser, CeraVe Hydrating Cleanser, and La Roche-Posay Toleriane Dermo-Cleanser.

Over-the-counter body cleanser suggestions include: Dove Sensitive Skin Unscented Beauty Bar, Aveeno Daily Moisturizing Body Wash, and Nature's Gate Purifying Liquid Soap.

Phase 2: Hydrate

I cannot overemphasize how critical hydration is. Skin dryness is the most common complaint among patients undergoing cancer treatment. Moisturizing your skin is important not only for your comfort but also for your overall health. If your skin is too dry, it can crack and become the source of opportunistic infections. To add moisture, you have to work from your head down to your toes, because every part of your body needs hydration.

There are two ways to moisturize your face. One is to use a serum, and the other is to apply a lotion or a cream. Some people prefer serums because, in general, they penetrate better. Others don't like them because some are sticky. If you choose a lotion or a cream, be sure to get one that has peptides or antioxidants. These are necessary to support your skin, which is being stressed by the chemicals of chemotherapy and targeted treatments.

The best time to add moisture to your body is right after your take a bath or a shower. After you have patted yourself off, slather on the moisturizer. When your skin is still a little damp, it absorbs moisturizers more effectively. Don't forget your feet and your hands. Apply concentrated healing moisture cream or balm that contains petrolatum or ceramides in an emollient base as a sealant.

Over-the-counter serum suggestions include: Lindi Skin Face Serum.

Over-the-counter facial moisturizer suggestions include: CeraVe Moisturizing Cream, Aveeno Ultra-Calming Daily Moisturizer with SPF 15, SkinCeuticals Hydrating B$_5$ Gel, Lindi Facial Lotion, and AVA MD Extreme Specialist Face Cream.

Over-the-counter body moisturizer suggestions include: Vaseline Body Lotion with Vitamin E and Aloe Vera, Origins Body Butter, and La Roche-Posay Toleriane Body Lotion.

Over-the-counter hand and foot cream suggestions include: Vanicream Moisturizing Skin Cream, Neutrogena Norwegian Formula Hand Cream, Neutrogena Norwegian Formula Cracked Heel Moisturizing Treatment, and Lindi Soothing Balm.

Phase 3: Get Complete UV Protection

Cancer treatment will make your skin particularly susceptible to damage from UVA and UVB rays, so it is more critical than ever to make sure that you never leave your home without applying a full-spectrum sunblock on all exposed areas. During cancer treatment you may find that your sunscreen is too irritating. In that case, use a physical sunblock (such as a mineral-based powder) or perhaps a sunblock designed for children. Actual physical protection —a hat, sunglasses, and sun-protective clothing—is also extremely important. Sun-protective clothing is available at sporting goods stores and online. You can add SPF protection to clothing by using a rinse in your wash, such as Rit Sun Guard.

Over-the-counter facial sunscreen suggestions include: EltaMD Skincare UV Physical SPF 41, Neutrogena Age Shield Face Sunblock, and Aveeno Ultra-Calming Daily Moisturizer.

Over-the-counter hand and body sunscreen suggestions include: Neutrogena Fresh Cooling Sunblock Gel SPF 45, EltaMD Skincare UV Physical SPF 41, and Eucerin Everyday Protection Body Lotion SPF 15.

Phase 4: Reapply

Reapply hydrating cream and full-spectrum UVA-UVB sunblock on all exposed areas, and cream or balm on the hands and the feet throughout the day. You can never use too much. A hydrophilic mist can provide extra hydration for your face and any dry area.

Over-the-counter suggestions include: AVA MD Antioxidant Mist and Avene Spray.

Rejuvenating Your Skin during Cancer Treatment

It is shocking to receive a diagnosis of cancer, with the prospect of chemotherapy, surgery, and radiation. It might seem frivolous to some, but my patients often want to have in-office rejuvenation treatments before their cancer therapy begins because it allows them to have control over one extremely important part of their physical and psychic well-being: how they look. Knowing that their appearance can be maintained, or at least retrieved at the end of treatment, is incredibly reassuring to them. Without exception, my patients tell me how grateful they are to be alive when so many others didn't make it. But they want to return to their lives looking their very best.

Here's what my patients want to know:

Can I continue to get hydrating facials during my cancer treatment?

Depending on your general health, your doctor may permit you to continue receiving gentle, moisturizing facials to fight the additional dryness brought on by chemotherapy. With their oncologists' permission, many of my patients benefit from home or professional facials during cancer treatment. There are aestheticians specifically trained to treat oncology patients. In general:

- Do not do extractions, exfoliation, or other procedures that might damage fragile skin.
- Use only the mildest products that are free of irritants and potential allergens.
- If your oncologist permits professional facials, have them performed in your dermatologist's office by a licensed aesthetician working under strict sanitary conditions.

- Always tell your dermatologist or aesthetician that you are undergoing cancer treatment before scheduling facials or other cosmetic treatments.

Should I even be thinking about rejuvenation while I'm having chemotherapy?

That's really a personal decision. For some of my patients, it's a huge priority; for others, not at all. Right now, your health and comfort are your first concern. If you still want to consider having a procedure, you and your dermatologist must get permission from your oncologist.

What can I do about the lines and wrinkles that have become so much more pronounced since I began chemotherapy?

The rapid acceleration of lines and wrinkles is a common, if unfortunate, side effect of chemotherapy as a result of dryness, stress on the skin, weight loss and gain, and premature menopause. We have many options for filling lines and restoring overall volume to the face to achieve a natural, healthy look. You will probably need to wait until your treatment is complete, however.

What can I do about the dark circles under my eyes?

For now, you wait and break out the concealer and the sunglasses. After you have recovered, there are many options that can erase them that include revolumizing the under-eye hollow and using skin lighteners.

I've finished my cancer treatment, but the skin on my face still has dark spots that appeared during treatment. Is there something I can do to get rid of them?

What you are describing is a common condition called post-inflammatory hyperpigmentation. Your dermatologist may prescribe a cream that contains a bleaching agent such as hydroquinone. It usually takes several months to see improvement. To help eliminate it, always use a sunscreen, because sun exposure can cause the spots to get darker. In the meantime, dark spots can be covered with makeup such as Dermablend.

Dr. Wendy's Eating Well during Cancer Treatment

Before Treatment

The time from first diagnosis to beginning treatment can feel like forever. Whether it's a week or a month, you're probably motivated to do just about anything to get yourself ready for treatment. That's exactly what you should do! One of the most important steps you can take to not only survive but to thrive is to eat well. It will help you set up a strong defense and boost your inner resources.

Even before diagnosis, there is a chance that you may experience some nutritional gaps or insufficiencies. Or you may just feel that your diet was not as good as it could be due to the regular stresses of daily living. This is the time to give yourself a boost. In fact, it's one thing you *can* do while you wait and prepare for treatment. Taking charge and getting ready for treatment is an empowering and important way of letting yourself (and the cancer) know that you are in control.

Although a diet that steers clear of processed and refined foods is always best, many people feel tempted to make radical shifts after diagnosis and explore the idea of trying all kinds of herbs and supplements. Keeping it simple is generally better. Depending on your time frame, getting your body ready means supporting its good health, not challenging it further. If you do choose to pursue some herbal formulas or supplements, seek advice from a trained and certified herbalist or a registered dietitian. And always get clearance from your oncologist first.

Health-Boosting Diet before Treatment
- Have a fruit or vegetable at every meal
- Lean protein at every meal—about 3–4 ounces (size of the palm of your hand)
- Whole grains in at least two of your three meals
- Soup or salad with lunch or dinner
- Two to three snacks—preferably fruits or vegetables
- 6–8 cups of water

- 3 cups fresh brewed green tea, spaced throughout the day (stop by 1 or 2 p.m. if you are sensitive to caffeine)
- Eat on a schedule, eating at similar times each day

Sample Menu

Day 1

Breakfast	Oatmeal with almonds, raisins, and low-fat milk Cup of green tea
Mid-morning	Piece of fruit or cup of low-sodium vegetable juice
Lunch	Entrée salad with grilled chicken and veggies, olive oil and vinegar or other all-natural salad dressing Slice of whole-grain toast
Afternoon snack	2 tablespoons almonds and 2 tablespoons raisins
Dinner	Salmon with sautéed broccoli and brown rice

Day 2

Breakfast	Yogurt and fresh berries with a sprinkle of low-fat granola or Kashi cereal
Mid-morning	Piece of fruit or cup of low-sodium vegetable juice
Lunch	Whole-grain pita sandwich with tuna salad made with low-fat Greek yogurt, chopped celery nd apple, and sliced tomato and lettuce Cup of veggie soup
Afternoon snack	Small yogurt with blueberries
Dinner	Whole-grain pasta with turkey Bolognese sauce, sprinkled with oregano Side salad of spinach, sliced almonds, and mandarin oranges in a light vinaigrette

Nutritious snack options
- Carrots and hummus
- Walnuts and dried cherries

- 2 whole-grain crackers with 1 tablespoon almond butter
- Sliced apple and 1 tablespoon peanut butter
- Blueberries and ½ cup fat-free or low-fat yogurt
- ½ half banana and a cup of fat-free or low-fat milk

Preparing for Chemotherapy

Anticipate some of the possibilities that may occur during treatment, and have your nutritional resources set and ready.

1. Stock different varieties of healthy options to ensure you have something you can tolerate and that can provide the nutrition you need.
2. Have simple foods ready to heat or ready to eat with minimal fuss.
3. Ask someone to help with food shopping and/or preparation if needed.

Stocking the Pantry, Fridge, and Freezer
- Stock foods that are nutritious and tasty.
- Keep favorite foods on hand. Even if they are not the best for you in terms of nutrition, sometimes eating in general is more important.
  - Purchase single-serving options like applesauce cups, low-fat pudding cups, instant oatmeal packets, all-natural energy bars, and granola bars.
  - Freeze some easy meals and snacks you can reheat:
    - Soups
    - Muffins
    - Pancakes
    - Casseroles
    - Lasagna
  - Find a local restaurant or health food store that has fresh, healthy soups made daily and stock up on several to a whole week's worth in individual one-cup servings.
  - Keep fruits and veggies on hand—fresh, frozen, and in jars for variety.

DR. WENDY'S RULE

There are actually no definitive rules when it comes to eating right for cancer treatment. Every person's experience is unique. What is most important is maintaining your energy and allowing your body to do its job along with your cancer treatment.

- Whole grains and complex starches are easy to digest and often provide comfort along with fiber.
- Include healthy carbs in your diet: brown rice, whole-wheat couscous, quinoa, whole-wheat bread, and potatoes (for baking, boiling, or mashing).
- Keep some healthy simple grains, too, like organic white rice and pasta.
- Include dried fruits and nuts for snacking.
- Keep the ingredients for smoothies on hand: bananas, yogurt, and frozen berries.
- Items like Popsicles and ginger tea are also useful, especially if you are dealing with certain side effects of chemotherapy.

Kitchen Tools to Have on Hand
- 1-cup glass storage containers with lids that are nice enough to eat out of—minimizes dish-washing but makes eating still somewhat of an occasion
- Storage containers and resealable bags to prepare individual portions and store extras

Sun Protection in Your Meal

Heightened sensitivity to the sun's harmful rays may be a potential side effect of your upcoming treatment. Sunscreen should be a given along with preventive habits like covering up and staying out of the sun during peak hours, but did you know there are some edible "sunscreens," as well?

A number of studies point to powerful compounds—flavonoids and carotenoids—found in foods like green tea and tomatoes that may help provide UV protection (or photoprotection) for the skin from the inside out. Research out of Germany shows that patients consuming the equivalent of $\frac{1}{4}$ cup of tomato paste a day had significantly lower UV damage after 10 to 12 weeks. Start now by enjoying your tomatoes, tomato paste, and tomato sauce regularly. Enjoy them with a little healthy anti-inflammatory fat like olive oil, avocado, or walnuts. Healthy oils help you absorb those powerful compounds. However, don't forget your sunscreen!

- Plastic disposable/recyclable or bamboo utensils
- Straws
- Lovely bottles, mugs, glasses, and glass pitchers—to remind you to sip, sip, sip throughout the day to stay hydrated and to move the nutrients through your body
- Electric teakettle

During Treatment

POOR APPETITE/LOSS OF APPETITE

You may lose your appetite, be nauseated, or have changes in taste and smell during treatment. These can affect your desire to eat and result in weight loss. It's very important to keep your weight stable to minimize muscle loss and to help encourage healing. Here are some tips:

- **Eat more protein.** A few extra bites of chicken or fish during your day, a scrambled or hard-boiled egg, or an extra teaspoon or two of peanut butter in your sandwich can boost the protein. Adding a few calories can help preserve your immune system and lean muscle tissue.
- **Sip some calories.** Add 100 percent juice to your water, sip on a smoothie, or even add a real milkshake to your day. Some people worry about a milkshake's fat and sugar, but the goal is to get extra calories. Smoothies can offer great nutrition and plenty of calories in an appealing and easy-to-eat way.
- **Try nuts and nut butter.** Keep a couple bowls of nuts around and have just a few here and there between meals and snacks; or spread a teaspoon of peanut or almond butter on a small cracker or a slice of apple.
- **Eat all-natural energy bars and granola bars.** Even just a few bites can add extra calories—and maybe some protein and fiber— to your daily intake.
- **Freeze bananas and grapes.** They're great nutrition, and changing the temperature and texture of healthy fruits is another way to add a few extra calories to your day.

- **Eat your favorite foods.** Have a little more of what is generally on the "watch out" list for nutrition—extra cheese on your salad or pasta, sour cream on your potato, and olive oil on your veggies.
- **Have comfort foods handy.** When the foods you enjoy are available, you may be more inclined to take a spoonful and get the calories you need. Grains like whole-grain toast or rice or oatmeal can be easy to digest and a good way to get some extra nutritious calories. Starchy vegetables like potatoes can be easy and helpful, too.
- **Eat more frequently.** Keep to a more frequent eating schedule. Eat every two hours instead of every three. Or make it a goal to have a few nuts every couple of hours until bedtime. Try to make it a bit of a game to add more eating to your day.
- **Never take or add any nutritional or herbal supplements to your diet unless your doctor has specifically approved it.**

SAMPLE CHEMO-DAY DIET

Before you go in for chemotherapy, it's important to have a good, solid base of nutrition in your system. Foods that are nutritious and well-tolerated work best. Here's a sample

Breakfast
- Slice of toast with peanut butter and banana
- Cup of green tea

Mid-morning
- Hard-boiled egg and some melon

Lunch
- Vegetable minestrone soup
- Half-sandwich with turkey, tomato, and lettuce

Afternoon snack
- Small yogurt and 15–20 grapes

Dinner
- Baked chicken, mashed potatoes, and cooked carrots

Evening Snack (optional)

- Ginger cookie
- Cup of herbal tea

WEIGHT GAIN

Some people experience weight gain during treatment. It's not uncommon, so don't despair. Weight gain can be caused by medications, reduction in physical activity, and fluid retention, among other reasons. If you gain a size or two, it's important to be smart and not try any drastic approaches to weight loss. Maintaining your health is always your first priority. The safest way to lose weight is to do it slowly and steadily by fueling weight loss with good food choices. Check with your oncologist before starting a weight-loss regimen. If approved, aim for a one- to two-pound weight loss weekly until you hit your goal.

- **Watch the empty calories.** These come from foods that offer calories—usually from sugar—but little else. Sugary drinks, candy, and cookies are examples.
- **Pay attention to portions.** Focus on eating high-nutrient, lower-calorie vegetables and fruits, modest lean proteins and grains, and less fats and empty calories overall. In general, your plate should be half veggies and fruits, a quarter lean protein, and a quarter whole grains.
- **Eat on a schedule.** Many times during treatment, people get off a regular schedule, eating around appointments or when they feel up to it. Get back on a regular eating routine of three meals and two to three snacks.
- **Don't skip meals.** To maintain your health and lose weight in the safest, most effective way, eat to fuel your metabolism. Skipping meals can mean skipping important nutrition, and it may set off cravings and the tendency to overeat later.
- **Keep a food diary.** Write down the time, meal, food, amount, and preparation technique. Also track your hunger level and mood. Be aware of what triggers you to eat and see if you can explore alternate ways to cope besides food. When you are hungry, eat nutritiously. When you are not, take a pause and let your body heal in other ways.

SENSITIVITY TO ODORS

Cancer treatment can affect not only your sense of taste but also your sense of smell, making it more difficult to consume food. To minimize unfavorable smells and maximize your ability to get the nutrition you need, follow these practices:

- Use a straw for fluids
- Keep foods cool
- Keep the house temperature a bit cooler and wear warmer clothes
- Open a window (if it's not too cold outside)
- Have food prepared outside of the house
- Don't eat where the food is prepared

DEHYDRATION

Nausea may prevent you from feeling like you can keep anything down, including water, but water is exactly what your body needs, especially if your skin, lips, or mouth become dry. Remember, you can eat your water, too. Use broths, vegetable juices, Popsicles, and juicy fruits like watermelon, and sip on tea, water, or other liquids you can tolerate.

Keep bottles, a thermos for drinks or soups, juice boxes, glasses, and pitchers handy so you have many ways to keep hydrated. Cold fluids have less aroma to them and therefore may be easier to tolerate when you're nauseous. Sipping through a straw may further help keep the aromas that can trigger nausea at bay.

METALLIC TASTE

Many women and men undergoing chemotherapy find that everything seems to take on a metallic taste. And it's worsened when you put that bite of food on your stainless-steel fork or spoon and into your mouth. One of the simplest changes you can make right away is to eat with disposable/recyclable plastic or reusable bamboo utensils. It may not completely take care of the changes in taste you experience, but it is guaranteed to make things taste a whole lot more like food and less like metal!

When you use plastic or bamboo utensils, make sure they are dishwasher safe or hand-wash thoroughly with dish detergent to keep them clean and safe for reuse.

Top Food Strategies for Good Energy

- **Sip, sip, sip.** Use a straw to reduce aromas and to keep your hydration steady and constant throughout the day. Stay hydrated with water, tea, soups, broths, and smoothies.
- **Have different textures available.** Sometimes you'll feel like something crunchy, sometimes like something chewy, and sometimes only liquids will do the trick.
- **Eat *something*.** Don't worry so much about "what"; eat what you can tolerate and what gives you more energy and less aggravation.
- **Keep it simple.** Your body wants to focus on healing, not fussing with food preparation. Eat nutritious foods but don't be afraid of convenience or enlisting help from others to prepare food that's easy to eat or reheat and eat.

WHEN NAUSEA STRIKES . . .

Nausea is a very common side effect of chemotherapy. While there are medications your doctor may prescribe for vomiting, feelings of nausea tend to nag because they continue for a longer period of time. So, try these strategies:

- **Keep it cool.** Cooler foods have less aroma than warm foods and will blunt the sensory response that might bring on feelings of nausea.
- **Eat smaller amounts**, but more frequently.
- **Eat away from where you cook.** The mixing of aromas from different ingredients combined with heat may increase the likelihood of nausea.
- **Go bland.** Strong flavors may enhance feelings of nausea.
- **Embrace your comfort zone.** Comfort foods come in handy when you're feeling uneasy. Mashed potatoes, toast, or other comfort foods can help.
- **Take your time.** Slow down your eating and drinking, and you may be able to calm the response of your stomach.
- **Rinse your mouth** and brush your teeth between meals to clear flavors and to reduce the chance of nausea.

- **Eat gingerly.** Recent research from the University of Rochester Medical Center showed that as little as ¼–½ teaspoon of ginger can significantly reduce the symptoms of nausea associated with chemotherapy. To add ginger to your diet: sip ginger tea, sprinkle ginger over fresh fruit, eat a ginger cookie, add ginger and cinnamon to morning oatmeal, grind ginger into squash or pumpkin soup, or use fresh ginger in marinades for chicken and fish.

After Treatment

Now is the time to make everything you've gone through really count. You may be tempted to celebrate and indulge in all the treats you feel you have missed out on during treatment. By all means, celebrate! But also get back to the basics so you can regain and rebuild your best health.

Those basics should include three meals and two to three snacks a day, eaten on a schedule. Practice portion control and eat mindfully. Your "forever" diet should include:

- Fruits, vegetables, beans, nuts, and seeds
- Healthy fats from fish, fish oils, olive oil, nuts, ground flaxseed, and avocados
- Lean proteins like fish and skinless turkey or chicken
- Whole grains
- 2–3 cups of green tea daily
- 8–10 cups of water daily
- Selective and special treats
- Moderate consumption of alcohol: 1 glass daily

If you've had some ups and downs when it came to eating as you went through treatment for cancer, your relationship with food may have suffered. Reintroduce the experience of dining by having fun with food.

- Sign up for an organic food co-op that delivers a "surprise" selection of local, seasonal foods on a weekly basis.

- Subscribe to a food or cooking-inspired magazine like *Eating Well* or *Cooking Light* and try a new recipe each week.
- Take a cooking class with a friend. Learn pasta techniques, how to make sushi, or the art of chocolate.
- Throw a dinner party with a theme. Choose an ethnic cuisine or make it an Iron Chef theme where everyone has to come with a selected course featuring a chosen ingredient.
- Volunteer for a few hours at a soup kitchen serving others nourishing meals.

Alisa's Fitness Tips

Oncologists used to caution cancer patients against physical activity for fear that it would only increase the fatigue caused by the disease and its treatment. Recent research, however, points to the critical importance of staying as physically active as you can before, during, and after your treatment.

Studies show that moderate exercise reduces the level of cytokines—chemical markers of inflammation—in the bloodstream. Reducing inflammation can help your body to turn its immune resources against the cancer cells and not the healthy tissues.

Obviously, getting fit and staying fit is also one of the best things you can do to improve your long-term prognosis. A Cambridge University study suggests that people who make healthy lifestyle choices are only one-fourth as likely to die from cancer or cardiovascular disease as those who don't make such choices. In an Ohio State University study, women treated for Stage II breast cancer with surgery and conventional chemotherapy and radiation were tracked for several years. Those who initiated simple lifestyle changes, such as practicing good nutrition and adding physical activity, were 68 percent less likely to die from a recurrence of their cancer within eleven years than those who did not make such changes. Exercise has been shown to reduce the recurrence of Stage III colon cancer by 40 to 50 percent.

There is so much that seems beyond your control when you are dealing with cancer. Doing what you can to stay active and fit is one way you can take the fight for healing into your own hands.

Skin Care Regimens during Cancer Treatment

OILY SKIN

MORNING REGIMEN

Step	Directions
Cleanse	Wash your face with a nondetergent, sulfate-free cleanser. *Note:* Use a cleanser designed for sensitive skin. If you need to exfoliate, mix your cleanser with half a teaspoon of baking soda.
Eyes	Gently dot a small amount of cream around the eyes. Choose products with ingredients that address your areas of concern. Vitamin K, caffeine, vitamin C, yarrow, horse chestnut, and gingko biloba address dark circles. Haloxyl, caffeine, vitamin C, cucumber extract, green tea, and aloe vera address puffiness. Hyaluronic acid, silica, soy proteins, acai berry, aloe vera, seaweed extracts, GABA, retinol, and argireline address wrinkles, firmness, and elasticity.
Moisturize	Every day: Apply a small amount of a light, oil-free, non-comedogenic moisturizer with anti-oxidants. If you have additional skin care needs: Choose an oil-free moisturizer with ingredients designed to address your specific skin care issues. Salicylic acid, azelaic acid, tea tree oil, and AHA address oil production and breakouts. Mulberry extract, arbutin, bearberry extract, licorice extract, kojic acid, azelaic acid, and gallic acid address sun damage and brown spots. Green tea, calendula, cucumber, aloe vera, chamomile, thyme, willow herb, perilla leaf extract, feverfew, red clove, evening primrose oil, zinc, mallow, red algae, silymarin, and ginger address inflammation and redness. Retinol, AHA, alpha-lipoic acid, basil, coenzyme Q10, hyaluronic acid, pomegranate, DMAE, lactic acid, caffeine, copper peptide, ferulic acid, grape seed extract, phytic acid, vitamin C, vitamin E, ursolic acid, silymarin, ginger, and ginseng address wrinkles.
Protect	Apply an oil-free, non-comedogenic sunblock every day. *Note:* If your skin doesn't tolerate sunblock, try a physical sunblock. It is organic and comes in a light powder form.

EVENING REGIMEN

Step	Directions
Cleanse	Wash your face with a nondetergent, sulfate-free cleanser. *Note:* Use a cleanser designed for sensitive skin.

Eyes	Gently dot a small amount of cream around the eyes. Choose products with ingredients that address your areas of concern. Vitamin K, caffeine, vitamin C, yarrow, horse chestnut, and gingko biloba address dark circles. Haloxyl, caffeine, vitamin C, cucumber extract, green tea, and aloe vera address puffiness. Retinol, hyaluronic acid, silica, soy proteins, acai berry, aloe vera, seaweed extracts, GABA, and argireline address wrinkles, firmness, and elasticity.
Moisturize	Every evening:

Apply a small amount of a light, oil-free, non-comedogenic moisturizer. If your skin is very sensitive, look for a hydrating, soothing, calming gel-type moisturizer.

If you have additional skin care needs:

Choose an oil-free moisturizer with ingredients designed to address your specific skin care issues. Salicylic acid, azelaic acid, tea tree oil, and AHA address oil production and breakouts. Mulberry extract, arbutin, bearberry extract, licorice extract, kojic acid, azelaic acid, and gallic acid address sun damage and brown spots. Green tea, calendula, cucumber, aloe vera, chamomile, thyme, willow herb, perilla leaf extract, feverfew, red clove, evening primrose oil, zinc, mallow, red algae, silymarin, and ginger address inflammation and redness. Retinol, AHA, alpha-lipoic acid, basil, coenzyme Q10, hyaluronic acid, pomegranate, DMAE, lactic acid, caffeine, copper peptide, ferulic acid, grape seed extract, phytic acid, vitamin C, vitamin E, ursolic acid, silymarin, ginger, and ginseng address wrinkles.

INGREDIENTS TO AVOID

If your skin is excessively oily: Mineral oil, petrolatum, coconut oil

If your skin is highly sensitive: Lactic acid, glycolic acid, alpha-lipoic acid, acetic acid, benzoic acid, cinnamic acid, menthol, parabens, quaternium-15, vitamin C

If you have existing discoloration: Celery extract, lime extract, parsley extract, fig extract, carrot extract, bergamot oil, estradiol, genistein

If your skin is acne-prone: Butyl stearate, cinnamon oil, isostearyl isostearate, cocoa butter, jojoba oil, coconut oil, decyl oleate, myristyl myristate, myristyl propionate, octyl palminate, octyl stearate, peppermint oil, isopropyl stearate, isopropyl isostearate, myristate, palmitate

AT-HOME TREATMENTS

You can purchase over-the-counter masks and exfoliates for oily skin, or you can make your own (see chapter 11).

Masks	You can apply a mask once or twice a week to tighten the pores and temporarily reduce excessive oil production. Masks are also helpful in reducing inflammation from acne flares.

Exfoliation	As long as your skin is relatively calm, you can use a gentle exfoliating scrub once a week. If you are experiencing a flare-up of acne or excessive oil production, do not use *any* kind of scrub.

COMBINATION SKIN

MORNING REGIMEN

Step	Directions
Cleanse	Wash with a gentle nondetergent, sulfate-free cleanser. *Note:* Use a cleanser designed for sensitive skin.
Eyes	Gently dot a small amount of cream around the eyes. Choose products with ingredients that address your areas of concern. Vitamin K, caffeine, vitamin C, yarrow, horse chestnut, and gingko biloba address dark circles. Haloxyl, caffeine, vitamin C, cucumber extract, green tea, and aloe vera address puffiness. Retinol, hyaluronic acid, silica, soy proteins, acai berry, aloe vera, seaweed extracts, GABA, and argireline address wrinkles, firmness, and elasticity.
Moisturize	Every day: Apply hydrating lotion with antioxidants. If you have additional skin care needs: Choose a moisturizer with ingredients designed to address your specific skin care issues. Azelaic acid, salicylic acid, glycolic acid, tea tree oil, and zinc address oil production and breakouts. Hyaluronic acid, ceramide, olive oil, dexpanthenol (provitamin B_5), evening primrose oil, borage seed oil, colloidal oatmeal, apricot kernel oil, macadamia nut oil, safflower oil, and jojoba oil address hydration. Kojic acid, mulberry extract, vitamin C, pine bark extract, strawberry begonia, and magnesium ascorbyl phosphate address sun damage and brown spots. Aloe vera, green tea, calendula, cucumber, thyme, chamomile, willow herb, perilla leaf extract, feverfew, evening primrose oil, red clove, mirabilis, colloidal oatmeal, red algae, and zinc address irritation and redness. Retinol, caffeine, green tea extract, coenzyme Q10 (ubiquinone), carrot extract, rosemary, grape seed extract, genistein, caffeine, copper peptide, ferulic acid, lutein, rosemary, basil, ginkgo biloba, and vitamin C address wrinkles. Azelaic acid, salicylic acid, tea tree oil, and zinc address acne flares.
Protect	Apply a chemical-free sunblock every day. You can use a sunblock designed to protect babies. *Note:* If your skin doesn't tolerate sunblock, try a physical sunblock. It is organic and comes in a light powder form.

EVENING REGIMEN

Step	Directions
Cleanse	Wash your face with a gentle nondetergent, sulfate-free cleanser. *Note:* Use a cleanser designed for sensitive skin.
Eyes	Gently dot a small amount of cream around the eyes. Choose products with ingredients that address your areas of concern. Vitamin K, caffeine, vitamin C, yarrow, horse chestnut, and gingko biloba address dark circles. Haloxyl, caffeine, vitamin C, cucumber extract, green tea, and aloe vera address puffiness. Retinol, hyaluronic acid, silica, soy proteins, acai berry, aloe vera, seaweed extracts, GABA, and argireline address wrinkles, firmness, and elasticity.
Moisturize	Every evening: Apply a light moisturizing lotion with ceramides and peptides. If you have additional skin care needs: Choose a moisturizer with ingredients designed to address your specific skin care issues. Azelaic acid, salicylic acid, glycolic acid, tea tree oil, and zinc address oil production and breakouts. Hyaluronic acid, ceramide, olive oil, dexpanthenol (provitamin B_5), evening primrose oil, borage seed oil, colloidal oatmeal, apricot kernel oil, macadamia nut oil, safflower oil, and jojoba oil address hydration. Kojic acid, mulberry extract, vitamin C, pine bark extract, strawberry begonia, and magnesium ascorbyl phosphate address sun damage and brown spots. Aloe vera, green tea, calendula, cucumber, thyme, chamomile, willow herb, perilla leaf extract, feverfew, evening primrose oil, red clove, mirabilis, colloidal oatmeal, red algae, and zinc address irritation and redness. Retinol, caffeine, green tea extract, coenzyme Q10 (ubiquinone), carrot extract, rosemary, grape seed extract, genistein, copper peptide, ferulic acid, lutein, rosemary, basil, ginkgo biloba, and vitamin C address wrinkles. Azelaic acid, salicylic acid, tea tree oil, and zinc address acne flares.

INGREDIENTS TO AVOID

If your skin is excessively oily: Mineral oil, petrolatum, coconut oil

If your skin is highly sensitive: Lactic acid, glycolic acid, alpha lipoic acid, acetic acid, benzoic acid, cinnamic acid, menthol, parabens, quaternium-15, vitamin C

If you have existing discoloration: Celery extract, lime extract, parsley extract, fig extract, carrot extract, bergamot oil, estradiol, genistein

If your skin is acne-prone: Butyl stearate, cinnamon oil, isostearyl isostearate, cocoa butter, jojoba oil, coconut oil, decyl oleate, myristyl myristate, myristyl propionate, octyl palminate, octyl stearate, peppermint oil, isopropyl stearate, isopropyl isostearate, myristate, palmitate

AT-HOME TREATMENTS

You can purchase over-the-counter masks and exfoliates for combination skin, or you can make your own (see chapter 11).

Masks	Your skin will benefit from using a mask once or twice a week to deliver hydration and a high concentration of nutrients.
Exfoliation	You may exfoliate once a week using a gentle natural exfoliant. If your skin is sensitive or has any issues like acne flares, don't exfoliate.

DRY SKIN

MORNING REGIMEN

Step	Directions
Cleanse	Wash with a gentle, soothing, nonfoaming, nondetergent, sulfate-free cleanser or use cold cream or facial cleansing oil. *Note:* Use a cleanser designed for sensitive skin.
Eyes	Gently dot a small amount of cream around the eyes. Choose products with ingredients that address your areas of concern. Vitamin K, caffeine, vitamin C, yarrow, horse chestnut, and gingko biloba address dark circles. Haloxyl, caffeine, vitamin C, cucumber extract, green tea, and aloe vera address puffiness. Retinol, hyaluronic acid, silica, soy proteins, acai berry, aloe vera, seaweed extracts, GABA, and argireline address wrinkles, firmness, and elasticity.
Moisturize	Every day: 　　While your skin is still damp, apply a moisturizer that contains moisture-locking ingredients like ceramides, peptides, and antioxidants. If you have additional skin care needs: 　　Choose a moisturizer with ingredients designed to address your specific skin care issues. Ceramide, borage seed oil, canola oil, apricot kernel oil, cocoa butter (don't use if you have acne), dexpanthenol, olive oil, glycerin, evening primrose oil, jojoba oil, macadamia nut oil, shea butter, safflower oil, colloidal oatmeal, dimethicone, lanolin (don't use if you have acne), and pumpkinseed oil address hydration. Green tea, calendula, cucumber, aloe vera, chamomile, feverfew, colloidal oatmeal, aloe vera, and thyme address redness and irritation. Arbutin, bearberry, cocos nucifera, cucumber extract, willow herb, gallic acid, kojic acid, vitamin C, mulberry extract, and pycnogenol (pine bark extract) address sun damage and brown spots. Salicylic acid, azelaic acid, and tea tree oil address acne flares (precede with moisturizer if skin is very dry). Retinol,

AHA, basil, lutein, lycopene, citric acid, lactic acid, phytic acid, polyhydroxy acid, carrot extract, rosemary, grape seed extract, genistein, caffeine, copper peptide, ferulic acid, and DMAE address wrinkles.

Protect	Apply chemical-free sunblock every day. You can use a sunblock designed to protect babies. *Note:* If your skin doesn't tolerate sunblock, try a physical sunblock. It is organic and comes in a light powder form.

EVENING REGIMEN

Step	Directions
Cleanse	Wash with a gentle, soothing, nonfoaming, nondetergent, sulfate-free cleanser or use cold cream or facial cleansing oil. *Note:* Use a cleanser designed for sensitive skin.
Eyes	Gently dot a small amount of cream around the eyes. Choose products with ingredients that address your areas of concern. Vitamin K, caffeine, vitamin C, yarrow, horse chestnut, and gingko biloba address dark circles. Haloxyl, caffeine, vitamin C, cucumber extract, green tea, and aloe vera address puffiness. Retinol, hyaluronic acid, silica, soy proteins, acai berry, aloe vera, seaweed extracts, GABA, and argireline address wrinkles, firmness, and elasticity.
Moisturize	Every evening: While your skin is still damp, apply a moisturizer that contains moisture-locking ingredients like ceramides and peptides. If you have additional skin care needs: Choose a moisturizer with ingredients designed to address your specific skin care issues. Ceramide, borage seed oil, canola oil, apricot kernel oil, cocoa butter (don't use if you have acne), dexpanthenol, olive oil, glycerin, evening primrose oil, jojoba oil, macadamia nut oil, shea butter, safflower oil, colloidal oatmeal, dimethicone, lanolin (don't use if you have acne), and pumpkinseed oil address hydration. Green tea, calendula, cucumber, aloe vera, chamomile, feverfew, colloidal oatmeal, aloe vera, and thyme address redness and irritation. Arbutin, bearberry, cocos nucifera, cucumber extract, willow herb, gallic acid, kojic acid, vitamin C, mulberry extract, and pycnogenol (pine bark extract) address sun damage and brown spots. Salicylic acid, azelaic acid, and tea tree oil address acne flares (precede with moisturizer if skin is very dry). Retinol, AHA, basil, lutein, lycopene, citric acid, lactic acid, phytic acid, polyhydroxy acid, carrot extract, rosemary, grape seed extract, genistein, caffeine, copper peptide, ferulic acid, and DMAE address wrinkles.

INGREDIENTS TO AVOID

If your skin is highly sensitive: Alcohol, lactic acid, glycolic acid, alpha-lipoic acid, acetic acid, benzoyl acid, cinnamic acid, polyhydroxy acid, phytic acid, vitamin C

If you have existing discoloration: Estradiol, estrogen, genistein, dandelion, geranium, jasmine, lavender, lemongrass, lemon oil, neroli oil, rose oil, tea tree oil, sandalwood

If your skin is acne-prone: Cinnamon oil, isotearyl isostearate, cocoa butter, coconut oil, peppermint oil, isopropyl myristate, isopropyl isostearate

AT-HOME TREATMENTS

You can purchase over-the-counter masks and exfoliates for dry skin, or you can make your own (see chapter 11). Don't use any type of exfoliation if you have existing irritations, rashes, or sores.

Masks	Masks can hydrate, reduce irritation, and soothe your skin. You can use a simple home-made mask (see chapter 11). If you have an acne or a rosacea flare, talk to your doctor before using a mask on your face or your body.
Exfoliation	Use only very gentle exfoliation at all times.

Skin Care Product List

Here are some additional over-the-counter skin care products that my patients like and that generally meet the requirements for gentleness during cancer treatment.

Cleansers

For the Face   Cetaphil Facial Cleanser
CeraVe Hydrating Cleanser
La Roche-Posay Toleriane Gentle
Dermo-Cleanser

For the Body   Dove Sensitive Skin Unscented Beauty Bar
Aveeno Daily Moisturizing Body Wash
Nature's Gate Purifying Liquid Soap
Lindi Skin Face Serum

Moisturizers

For the Face   CeraVe Moisturizing Cream
Aveeno Ultra-Calming Daily Moisturizer with SPF 15
SkinCeuticals Hydrating B_5 Gel
Lindi Facial Lotion
AVA MD Extreme Specialist Face Cream

For the Body   Vaseline Body Lotion with Vitamin E and Aloe Vera
Origins Body Butter
La Roche-Posay Toleriane Body Lotion
Vanicream Moisturizing Skin Cream
Neutrogena Norwegian Formula Hand Cream
Neutrogena Norwegian Formula Cracked Heel
   Moisturizing Treatment
Lindi Soothing Balm

Sun Protection

For the Face   Lindi Sun, Unscented
EltaMD Skincare UV Physical SPF 41
Neutrogena Age Shield FACE Sunblock

For the Body   Neutrogena Fresh Cooling Sunblock Gel SPF 45
EltaMD Skincare UV Physical SPF 41
Eucerin Everyday Protection Body Lotion SPF 15

Skin Care Regimens after Cancer Treatment

OILY SKIN

MORNING REGIMEN

Step	Directions
Cleanse	Wash with a nondetergent cleanser. A low percentage of glycolic acid may be one of the ingredients.
Tone	Mist with antioxidant facial water, if needed. You can use glycolic acid pads or oil-control gel on the T-zone, if needed, but don't overdry your face.

Serum	To add more nutrients to your skin, apply serum to rejuvenate, firm, and address other concerns. Alpha-lioic acid, coenzyme Q10 (ubiquinone), pomegranate, DMAE, lactic acid, caffeine, copper peptide, ferulic acid, phytic acid, vitamin C, basil, grape seed extract, lutein, lycopene, green tea, ginseng, genistein, silymarin, vitamin E, resveratrol, acai berry, AHA, retinol, and apple stem cell address rejuvenation.
Eyes	Gently dot a small amount of cream around the eyes. Choose products with ingredients that address your areas of concern. Vitamin K, caffeine, vitamin C, yarrow, horse chestnut, and gingko biloba address dark circles. Haloxyl, caffeine, vitamin C, cucumber extract, green tea, and aloe vera address puffiness. Retinol, hyaluronic acid, silica, soy proteins, acai berry, aloe vera, seaweed extracts, GABA, and argireline address wrinkles, firmness, and elasticity.

Moisturize	Every day:
	
	    Apply a small amount of oil-free moisturizer with ingredients like antioxidants, vitamins, and minerals.
	
	If you have additional skin care needs:
	
	    Choose an oil-free moisturizer with ingredients designed to treat your specific skin care issues. Salicylic acid, benzoyl peroxide, azelaic acid, tea tree oil, phytic acid, and peppermint oil address oil production and breakouts. Green tea, calendula, cucumber, aloe vera, chamomile, thyme, willow herb, perilla leaf extract, feverfew, red clove, evening primrose oil, zinc, mallow, red algae, silymarin, ginger, lavender, azulene, and blue lotus address inflammation and irritation. Hydroquinone, mulberry extract, niacinamide, arbutin, bearberry extract, licorice extract, kojic acid, azelaic acid, and gallic acid address brown spots. Retinol, AHA, alpha-lipoic acid, basil, coenzyme Q10, hyaluronic acid, pomegranate, DMAE, lactic acid, caffeine, copper peptide, ferulic acid, and grape seed extract address wrinkles.

Protect	Apply an oil-free, broad-spectrum, and non-comedogenic sunblock *every day.* *Note:* If your moisturizer contains a sunscreen of at least SPF 25 that blocks UVA and UVB rays, you don't need to add extra sunblock.

EVENING REGIMEN

Step	*Directions*
Cleanse	Wash with a nondetergent cleanser. A low percentage of glycolic acid or tea tree oil may be one of the ingredients.
Tone	If needed, gently wipe your face with toner or spray with facial water.
Serum	To add more nutrients to your skin, apply serum to rejuvenate, firm, and address other concerns. Alpha-lioic acid, coenzyme Q10 (ubiquinone), pomegranate, DMAE, lactic

acid, caffeine, copper peptide, ferulic acid, phytic acid, vitamin C, basil, grape seed extract, lutein, lycopene, green tea, ginseng, genistein, silymarin, vitamin E, resveratrol, acai berry, AHA, retinol, and apple stem cell address rejuvenation.

Eyes	Gently dot a small amount of cream around the eyes. Choose products with ingredients that address your areas of concern. Vitamin K, caffeine, vitamin C, yarrow, horse chestnut, and gingko biloba address dark circles. Haloxyl, caffeine, vitamin C, cucumber extract, green tea, and aloe vera address puffiless. Retinol, hyaluronic acid, silica, soy proteins, acai berry, aloe vera, seaweed extracts, GABA, and argireline address wrinkles, firmness, and elasticity.
Moisturize	Every evening: Apply a small amount of moisturizer with retinol. If you have additional skin care needs: Choose an oil-free moisturizer with ingredients designed to treat your specific skin care issues. Salicylic acid, benzoyl peroxide, azelaic acid, tea tree oil, phytic acid, and peppermint oil address oil production and breakouts. Green tea, calendula, cucumber, aloe vera, chamomile, thyme, willow herb, perilla leaf extract, feverfew, red clove, evening primrose oil, zinc, mallow, red algae, silymarin, ginger, lavender, azulene, and blue lotus address inflammation and irritation. Hydroquinone, mulberry extract, niacinamide, arbutin, bearberry extract, licorice extract, kojic acid, azelaic acid, and gallic acid address brown spots. Retinol, AHA, alpha-lipoic acid, basil, coenzyme Q10, hyaluronic acid, pomegranate, DMAE, lactic acid, caffeine, copper peptide, ferulic acid, and grape seed extract address wrinkles.

INGREDIENTS TO AVOID

If your skin is excessively oily: Mineral oil, petrolatum, coconut oil

If your skin is highly sensitive: Lactic acid, glycolic acid, alpha-lipoic acid, acetic acid, benzoic acid, cinnamic acid, menthol, parabens, quaternium-15, vitamin C

If you have existing discoloration: Celery extract, lime extract, parsley extract, fig extract, carrot extract, bergamot oil, estradiol, genistein

If your skin is acne-prone: Butyl stearate, cinnamon oil, isostearyl isostearate, cocoa butter, jojoba oil, coconut oil, decyl oleate, myristyl myristate, myristyl propionate, octyl palminate, octyl stearate, peppermint oil, isopropyl stearate, isopropyl isostearate, myristate, palmitate

AT-HOME TREATMENTS

You can purchase over-the-counter masks and exfoliates for oily skin, or you can make your own (see chapter 11).

| Masks | You can apply a mask once or twice a week to tighten the pores and temporarily reduce excessive oil production. Masks are also helpful in reducing inflammation from acne flares. |
| Exfoliation | As long as your skin is relatively calm, you can use a gentle exfoliating scrub once a week. If you are experiencing a flare-up of acne or excessive oil production, do not use any kind of scrub. |

COMBINATION SKIN

MORNING REGIMEN

Step	Directions
Cleanse	Wash with a nonsoap cleanser that contains polyhydroxy acid.
Tone	Gently wipe your face with a hydrating toner or spray with antioxidant mist. You can use glycolic acid pads or oil-control gel on the T-zone, if needed, but don't overdry your face.
Serum	To add more nutrients to your skin, apply serum to rejuvenate, firm, and address other concerns. Alpha-lioic acid, coenzyme Q10 (ubiquinone), pomegranate, DMAE, lactic acid, caffeine, copper peptide, ferulic acid, phytic acid, vitamin C, basil, grape seed extract, lutein, lycopene, green tea, ginseng, genistein, silymarin, vitamin E, resveratrol, acai berry, AHA, retinol, and apple stem cell address rejuvenation.
Eyes	Gently dot a small amount of cream around the eyes. Choose products with ingredients that address your areas of concern. Vitamin K, caffeine, vitamin C, yarrow, horse chest-nut, and gingko biloba address dark circles. Haloxyl, caffeine, vitamin C, cucumber extract, green tea, and aloe vera address puffiness. Retinol, hyaluronic acid, silica, soy proteins, acai berry, aloe vera, seaweed extracts, GABA, and argireline address wrinkles, firmness, and elasticity.

Moisturize	Every day:
	    Apply a small amount of moisturizer with antioxidants.
	If you have additional skin care needs:
	    Choose a moisturizer with ingredients designed to treat your specific skin care issues. Azelaic acid, salicylic acid, glycolic acid, tea tree oil, and zinc address oil production and breakouts. Hyaluronic acid, ceramide, olive oil, dexpanthenol (provitamin B_5), evening primrose oil, borage seed oil, colloidal oatmeal, apricot kernel oil, borage seed oil, macadamia nut oil, safflower oil, and jojoba oil address hydration. Niacinamide, kojic

acid, mulberry extract, vitamin C, pine bark extract, strawberry begonia, and magnesium ascorbyl phosphate address brown spots. Aloe vera, green tea, calendula, cucumber, thyme, chamomile, willow herb, perilla leaf extract, feverfew, evening primrose oil, red clove, mirabilis, colloidal oatmeal, red algae, and zinc address irritation and inflammation. Retinol, caffeine, green tea extract, coenzyme Q10 (ubiquinone), carrot extract, rosemary, grape seed extract, genistein, copper peptide, ferulic acid, lutein, rosemary, basil, ginkgo biloba, and vitamin C address wrinkles. Azelaic acid, salicylic acid, tea tree oil, and zinc address acne flares.

Protect	Apply broad-spectrum sunblock *every day*.
	Note: If your moisturizer contains a sunscreen of at least SPF 25 that blocks UVA and UVB rays, you don't need to add extra sunblock.

EVENING REGIMEN

Step	*Directions*
Cleanse	Wash your face with a nondetergent cleanser.
Tone	Gently wipe your face with hydrating toner.
Serum	To add more nutrients to your skin, apply serum to rejuvenate, firm, and address other concerns. Alpha-lioic acid, coenzyme Q10 (ubiquinone), pomegranate, DMAE, lactic acid, caffeine, copper peptide, ferulic acid, phytic acid, vitamin C, basil, grape seed extract, lutein, lycopene, green tea, ginseng, genistein, silymarin, vitamin E, resveratrol, acai berry, AHA, retinol, and apple stem cell address rejuvenation.
Eyes	Gently dot a small amount of cream around the eyes. Choose products with ingredients that address your areas of concern. Vitamin K, caffeine, vitamin C, yarrow, horse chestnut, and gingko biloba address dark circles. Haloxyl, caffeine, vitamin C, cucumber extract, green tea, and aloe vera address puffiness. Retinol, hyaluronic acid, silica, soy proteins, acai berry, aloe vera, seaweed extracts, GABA, and argireline address wrinkles, firmness, and elasticity.
Moisturize	Every evening:
	Apply a small amount of a moisturizer with retinol. Be careful not to overdry or irritate your skin.
	If you have additional skin care needs:
	Choose an oil-free moisturizer with ingredients designed to treat your specific skin care issues. Azelaic acid, salicylic acid, glycolic acid, tea tree oil, and zinc address oil production and breakouts. Hyaluronic acid, ceramide, olive oil, dexpanthenol (provitamin B_5), evening primrose oil, borage seed oil, colloidal oatmeal, apricot kernel oil,

borage seed oil, macadamia nut oil, safflower oil, and jojoba oil address hydration. Niacinamide, kojic acid, mulberry extract, vitamin C, pine bark extract, strawberry begonia, and magnesium ascorbyl phosphate address brown spots. Aloe vera, green tea, calendula, cucumber, thyme, chamomile, willow herb, perilla leaf extract, feverfew, evening primrose oil, red clove, mirabilis, colloidal oatmeal, red algae, and zinc address irritation and inflammation. Retinol, caffeine, green tea extract, coenzyme Q10 (ubiquinone), carrot extract, rosemary, grape seed extract, genistein, copper peptide, ferulic acid, lutein, rosemary, basil, ginkgo biloba, and vitamin C address wrinkles. Azelaic acid, salicylic acid, tea tree oil, and zinc address acne flares.

INGREDIENTS TO AVOID

If your skin is excessively oily: Mineral oil, petrolatum, coconut oil

If your skin is highly sensitive: Lactic acid, glycolic acid, alpha-lipoic acid, acetic acid, benzoic acid, cinnamic acid, menthol, parabens, quaternium-15, vitamin C

If you have existing discoloration: Celery extract, lime extract, parsley extract, fig extract, carrot extract, bergamot oil, estradiol, genistein

If your skin is acne-prone: Butyl stearate, cinnamon oil, isostearyl isostearate, cocoa butter, jojoba oil, coconut oil, decyl oleate, myristyl myristate, myristyl propionate, octyl palminate, octyl stearate, peppermint oil, isopropyl stearate, isopropyl isostearate, myristate, palmitate

AT-HOME TREATMENTS

You can purchase over-the-counter masks and exfoliates for combination skin, or you can make your own (see chapter 11).

Masks	Your skin will benefit from using a mask once or twice a week to deliver hydration and high concentrations of nutrients.
Exfoliation	Using a fine-textured scrub, you may exfoliate once a week to remove the top layer of dead skin cells. Don't exfoliate if you have very sensitive skin or if your acne medication creates irritation.

IN-OFFICE PROCEDURES

Peel   Microdermabrasion   Cleansing and hydrating facial treatment

Laser treatment   Radio-frequency treatment.

DRY SKIN

MORNING REGIMEN

Step	Directions
Cleanse	Wash with a gentle, soothing, nonfoaming cleanser or use cold cream.
Tone	Mist your face with an antioxidant spray and follow quickly with the application of a hydrating serum.
Serum	To add more nutrients to your skin, apply serum to rejuvenate, firm, and address other concerns. Alpha-lioic acid, coenzyme Q10 (ubiquinone), pomegranate, DMAE, lactic acid, caffeine, copper peptide, ferulic acid, phytic acid, vitamin C, basil, grape seed extract, lutein, lycopene, green tea, ginseng, genistein, silymarin, vitamin E, resveratrol, acai berry, AHA, retinol, and apple stem cell address rejuvenation.
Eyes	Gently dot a small amount of cream around the eyes. Choose products with ingredients that address your areas of concern. Vitamin K, caffeine, vitamin C, yarrow, horse chestnut, and gingko biloba address dark circles. Haloxyl, caffeine, vitamin C, cucumber extract, green tea, and aloe vera address puffiness. Retinol, hyaluronic acid, silica, soy proteins, acai berry, aloe vera, seaweed extracts, GABA, and argireline address wrinkles, firmness, and elasticity.

Moisturize	Every day:
	    While your skin is still damp from the hydrating serum, apply moisturizer with antioxidants and ceramides.
	If you have additional skin care needs:
	    Choose a moisturizer with ingredients designed to treat your specific skin care issues. Ceramide, borage seed oil, canola oil, apricot kernel oil, cocoa butter (don't use if you have acne), dexpanthenol, olive oil, glycerin, evening primrose oil, jojoba oil, macadamia nut oil, shea butter, safflower oil, colloidal oatmeal, dimethicone, lanolin (don't use if you have acne), and pumpkinseed oil address hydration. Green tea, calendula, cucumber, aloe vera, chamomile, feverfew, colloidal oatmeal, aloe vera, and thyme address irritation and inflammation. Arbutin, bearberry, coconut palm, cucumber extract, willow herb, gallic acid, hydroquinone, kojic acid, vitamin C, mulberry extract, and pycnogenol (pine bark extract) address brown spots. AHA, basil, lutein, lycopene, citric acid, lactic acid, phytic acid, polyhydroxy acid, carrot extract, rosemary, grape seed extract, genistein, caffeine, copper peptide, ferulic acid, and DMAE address wrinkles. Salicylic acid, azelaic acid, benzoyl peroxide, and tea tree oil address acne flares (precede with moisturizer if skin is very dry).

Protect	Apply broad-spectrum sunblock *every day.*
	Note: If your moisturizer contains a sunscreen of at least SPF 25 that blocks UVA and UVB rays, you don't need to add extra sunblock.

EVENING REGIMEN

Step	Directions
Cleanse	Wash your face with a soap-free cleanser that contains calendula, chamomile, or other soothing ingredients.
Tone	Mist your face with a facial rosewater or hydrating toner.
Serum	To add more nutrients to your skin, apply serum to rejuvenate, firm, and address other concerns. Alpha-lioic acid, coenzyme Q10 (ubiquinone), pomegranate, DMAE, lactic acid, caffeine, copper peptide, ferulic acid, phytic acid, vitamin C, basil, grape seed extract, lutein, lycopene, green tea, ginseng, genistein, silymarin, vitamin E, resveratrol, acai berry, AHA, retinol, and apple stem cell address rejuvenation.
Eyes	Gently dot a small amount of cream around the eyes. Choose products with ingredients that address your areas of concern. Vitamin K, caffeine, vitamin C, yarrow, horse chestnut, and gingko biloba address dark circles. Haloxyl, caffeine, vitamin C, cucumber extract, green tea, and aloe vera address puffiness. Retinol, hyaluronic acid, silica, soy proteins, acai berry, aloe vera, seaweed extracts, GABA, and argireline address wrinkles, firmness, and elasticity.
Moisturize	Every evening:
	While your skin is still damp, apply a moisturizer that contains moisture-locking ingredients like ceramides and peptides.
	If you have additional skin care needs:
	Choose a moisturizer with ingredients designed to treat your specific skin care issues. Ceramide, borage seed oil, canola oil, apricot kernel oil, cocoa butter (don't use if you have acne), dexpanthenol, olive oil, glycerin, evening primrose oil, jojoba oil, macadamia nut oil, shea butter, safflower oil, colloidal oatmeal, dimethicone, lanolin (don't use if you have acne), and pumpkinseed oil address hydration. Green tea, calendula, cucumber, aloe vera, chamomile, feverfew, colloidal oatmeal, aloe vera, and thyme address irritation and inflammation. Arbutin, bearberry, coconut palm, cucumber extract, willow herb, gallic acid, hydroquinone, kojic acid, vitamin C, mulberry extract, and pycnogenol (pine bark extract) address brown spots. AHA, basil, lutein, lycopene, citric acid, lactic acid, phytic acid, polyhydroxy acid, carrot extract, rosemary, grape

seed extract, genistein, caffeine, copper peptide, ferulic acid, and DMAE address wrinkles. Salicylic acid, azelaic acid, benzoyl peroxide, retinol (for evening use only), and tea tree oil address acne flares (precede with moisturizer if skin is very dry).

INGREDIENTS TO AVOID

If your skin is highly sensitive: Alcohol, lactic acid, glycolic acid, alpha-lipoic acid, acetic acid, benzoyl acid, cinnamic acid, polyhydroxy acid, phytic acid, vitamin C

If you have existing discoloration: Estradiol, estrogen, genistein, dandelion, geranium, jasmine, lavender, lemongrass, lemon oil, neroli oil, rose oil, tea tree oil, sandalwood

If your skin is acne-prone: Cinnamon oil, isotearyl isostearate, cocoa butter, coconut oil, peppermint oil, isopropyl myristate, isopropyl isostearate

AT-HOME TREATMENTS

You can purchase over-the-counter masks and exfoliates for dry skin or you can make your own (see chapter 11).

Masks	Masks can hydrate, reduce irritation, and be very soothing. You can use a simple homemade mask or purchase one over the counter. Make sure when purchasing a mask that it is specifically made for sensitive skin and doesn't have any of the chemicals or ingredients that are listed above. If you have an acne or a rosacea flare, talk to your health care provider before using a mask on your face or your body.
Exfoliation	Use only very gentle facial exfoliates. Homemade scrubs are a good option. Make sure that the exfoliate doesn't contain any fragrance or other chemicals. If your skin is very sensitive, you can exfoliate with dry oatmeal. Do not use any peels or other microdermabrasion kits.

IN-OFFICE PROCEDURES

Cleansing and hydrating facial treatment   Laser treatment   Radio-frequency treatment

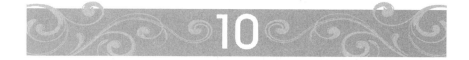

Restoring Your Skin through Fitness

Remember when you were a child and you would feel flushed after you spent the day sledding, making snowmen, or spending a day at the pool challenging your friends to see who could swim fastest to the other side? That's the wonderful glow of good health and good skin. As we get older, of course, things change. We don't eat as well as we should, we don't have as much time to exercise as we'd like, or we don't know how to exercise—and it shows on our skin.

It's never too late to start healing your skin, however, and one of the best ways to do that is by learning how to care for your body. In this chapter you will:

- Understand the connection between fitness and healthy skin
- Learn how fitness skills can help your skin through the challenges of adult acne, menopause, and serious illness
- Find fitness plans to incorporate into your skin-healing program

First take a minute to congratulate yourself. You're making a commitment to your fitness, and it always takes a great deal of courage to make a lifestyle change, but you are also taking a leap of faith in *yourself*. That's a marvelous and empowering step! Just remember to be patient. Achieving your long-term fitness goals is not simply a matter of going through the correct motions. It's also a lesson in learning to have patience. With consistency and commitment, you will get results. By results I mean the great, glowing, healthy skin you remember from your childhood.

The Skin Benefits of Fitness

In this section, I'll outline some of the direct benefits your skin receives from regular physical activity. I'll also provide a basic primer on the components of a multimodal fitness plan—the kind of diversified physical activity (such as aerobics, weight training, and yoga) that has been proven to offer the best results for skin and overall health. With the help of Alisa Daglio, a fitness expert who helped *Extreme Makeover* participants to become active and fit, I'll share some motivation strategies.

First and foremost, an effective fitness regimen is enjoyable. (Notice I didn't say *easy*.) It reduces stress, enhances circulation, improves nutrient delivery to skin cells, and can even modify hormonal shifts. All of these benefits directly improve the health and appearance of your skin.

Exercise can help you to overcome stress even when you can't avoid stressful situations. Countless studies have proven that almost every type of physical activity can have powerful stress-reduction effects. Vigorous exercise seems to signal to the brain that you're doing something productive to handle the stress (either fighting or fleeing), so it shuts down the stress hormones, regularizes the heart rate, and stops diverting oxygen and nutrients away from your skin.

Yoga, breathing, stretching, and disciplines like Tai Chi, though less vigorous, are also stress relievers. Regular exercise also promotes a healthy sleep cycle, which is vital to your skin's natural repair and renewal processes.

Exercise breaks the inflammation cycle in the body, calming and cooling your system. When your mind and your body are calmer, your skin is calmer. With regular exercise, you'll see less redness and inflammation, fewer blemishes, and a faster turnover of dead skin cells.

Muscles that are toned are better able to relax and be more elastic, which reduces the appearance of wrinkling and sagging. Exercise improves the efficiency of your circulatory system by delivering oxygen and nutrients to starved cells, keeping blood vessels flexible and unclogged by plaque, and stimulating digestive regularity. When you practice good fitness habits along with good nutrition, your skin will reward you with a healthy glow. The improved circulation that comes from physical fitness also promotes the ideal conditions for your cells to produce collagen and elastin, the proteins that give your skin its underlying structure, support, and resilience.

> **ALISA'S BODY SAVER**
>
> Low abdominal breathing is an excellent way to reduce stress. Inhale deeply through your nose while letting your lower abdomen fill like a balloon. Exhale through your mouth and contract your stomach muscles inward as you push the air out. This can help you to release stress, regulate your mood, and improve the look of your skin. An added bonus is that this form of breathing expedites weight loss by oxygenating the muscles properly and enabling you to burn more body fat.

The benefits of exercise don't apply just to what goes into your skin; they influence what comes out, too. Vigorous exercise works up a sweat, which helps to regulate body temperature as the sweat evaporates. When you sweat, your skin performs a valuable detoxification function. Through its network of pores, your skin is responsible for clearing out about 30 percent of the toxins and waste products that your body gets rid of every day.

Along with controlling stress hormones, physical activity helps to control other hormonal surges that can be harmful to your overall health and that of your skin. Studies show that when you exercise, your adrenal glands produce less DHT and DHEA, the hormones responsible in part for acne. Regular cardiovascular workouts, such as fast walking or moderate cycling, also inhibit the secretion of corticosteroids. Staying active has been proven to modify the fluctuations in sex hormones (testosterone and estrogen) that occur during puberty and around menopause and that trigger acne outbreaks and troublesome symptoms like hot flashes.

The Components of Total
Body Fitness

When Alisa and I worked on *Extreme Makeover*, we emphasized the importance of a multimodal approach, combining complementary techniques to achieve the best results in fitness and skin health. It worked very successfully for the *Extreme Makeover* participants, who were making big changes in their appearances in a very limited time frame. It will work for you as well, as you make a life-long commitment to healthier skin through fitness.

Variety is essential to a sustainable, whole-body fitness program in the same way that a varied diet is essential to a healthy body. In other words, you can't just do one exercise (or type of exercise) and expect to become fit. This section outlines the essential components of an effective fitness program. Alisa's sample four-day fitness regimen, which incorporates many of these elements, can be found later in this chapter.

Exercise that strengthens your cardiovascular system and improves your endurance is known as *cardio* or *aerobic* exercise. Aerobic exercise is physical activity that is carried out at a moderate level for an extended period. Regular aerobic exercise has the following benefits for the cardiovascular system:

- Strengthens the heart muscle so that it pumps more effectively
- Lowers blood pressure and the resting heart rate
- Improves circulation throughout the body
- Delivers oxygen to the cells more efficiently by strengthening the breathing muscles and by generating more of the red blood cells that transport oxygen
- Increases the basal metabolic rate, processing carbohydrates and fats and storing energy in your muscles to make them stronger

Cardio also reduces the risk of developing diabetes, heart disease, and stroke. High-impact aerobic exercise like running builds bone density. There are also many skin benefits: better circulation, lower inflammation,

ALISA'S BODY SAVER

Remember to consult your doctor before engaging in any new exercise regimen. Be sure to discuss any medications you are taking, because side effects can be triggered by, or can limit the effects of, exercise. When in doubt, start off slowly and build momentum.

and retained firmness and elasticity through stepped-up collagen production.

Cardio encompasses many popular forms of exercise and physical activities, including the following:

- Brisk walking, outdoors or on a treadmill
- Cycling, outdoors or on a stationary bike
- Swimming
- Running
- Rowing a boat or using a rowing machine
- Dancing, either informally or to popular hip-hop workouts or the Latin music workout known as Zumba
- Vigorous martial arts, like Tae Bo or kickboxing
- Jumping rope
- Cross-country skiing

There are many ways to incorporate aerobic exercise into your fitness routine, whether outdoors, at home, or in a gym. For maximum effectiveness, work cardio into your fitness routine three or four times a week. Start slowly—with as little as five minutes at a time if you haven't worked out in the past—and work up to your goal as you are able.

Whereas cardio training builds the strength of your internal systems, strength training builds your muscles by working them against force. Stronger muscles support and protect your bones and make it easier for you to move through all the activities of your day. Strength training manages blood sugar, reducing the need for insulin and storing energy in the muscles instead of in fatty tissues. It contributes to great-looking skin by toning the muscles to which the skin is attached.

You can strengthen your muscles through resistance training, in which you work your muscles against elastic bands or hydraulic exercise machines, or weight

ALISA'S BODY SAVER

Does the skin under your upper arm keep waving good-bye long after the rest of your arm has stopped? Tame loose upper-arm skin for good by performing the following isotonic exercise that focuses on the inner head of the triceps:

- Securely attach an exercise band with handles to a stable object at an angle.
- Bend your knees and keep your elbows tightly at your sides as your arm forms a ninety-degree angle (palms facing up).
- While keeping your shoulders back, pull the band handles downward until your arms become straight along the sides of your body.
- Keep your wrists locked backward and hold the position for two or three seconds.

training, which uses free weights or machines to add resistance. Most strength training is anaerobic because you are expending energy in short bursts. Strength training can have an aerobic quality if you build endurance by doing many repetitions. However, each repetition should be performed in a controlled manner, not in a jerky fashion.

Strengthening exercises come in two forms: *isometric* and *isotonic.* In isometric exercise, you contract a muscle without moving the joint. In isotonic exercise, you move your joints to push against the weight or resistance. Perform strength-training exercises every other day or work different muscle groups on different days. This will give your muscles time to rest and repair themselves in between sessions.

ALISA'S BODY SAVER

A lot of women worry that strength training will make them bulk up. Don't confuse strength training with body-building, in which the goal is to increase muscle size and definition. You may see your weight go up a little as you work with weights or resistance bands, but what you're seeing isn't added fat, it's denser muscle fiber. Your body will actually look leaner and more sculpted or toned. You may find that you actually lose inches and drop a clothing size as your muscles provide better support for your frame.

One area of strength training that's receiving a lot more attention lately is core training, or strengthening the muscles at the core of your body that support your spine and your abdomen. Core training combines muscle-strengthening exercises like abdominal crunches with activities designed to improve balance and stability. Pilates, which uses patented machines and devices like balance balls, is the best-known core-training system, but you can incorporate core stability work into any fitness routine. Deep-breathing exercises are the most effective abdominal exercise you can find. When performed correctly, you will contract the muscles all the way down to your pelvic floor.

Every fitness routine should include exercises to improve flexibility. Flexibility routines make muscles more elastic and resilient and allow stiff joints to move more freely.

Because most flexibility work involves gentle movement and coordinated deep breathing, it has a powerful stress-fighting effect and improves circulation and respiration. Flexibility routines help the skin by improving circulation, easing stress, and calming inflammation.

Many popular routines are derived from Eastern disciplines. Yoga and Tai Chi are the most commonly practiced. These disciplines employ a combination of stretching, programmed breathing, and held poses (yoga) or flowing movements with shifting balance (Tai Chi).

Flexibility routines also include simple stretches and range-of-motion exercises that gently work the joints and muscle groups without resistance.

Rest is also an essential part of a fitness program. Most of us do not get enough sleep (which is defined as eight hours a night), and it can greatly affect our overall health. Insufficient sleep has been linked to depression, increased risk of obesity, and numerous other health problems. Lack of sleep also does terrible things to your skin, because your skin—like all the other cells in your body—does its best healing and replenishing while you're asleep.

You need enough rest to make the other elements in your fitness regimen pay off. Studies of sleep-deprived athletes show that cardiovascular functioning weakens by more than 10 percent, glucose metabolism drops by up to 40 percent, and reaction times and muscle strength soon start to resemble those of elderly sedentary people. Here's another statistic to give you pause: sleep-deprived people consume 45 percent more carbohydrates than those who get adequate rest.

Consider a good night's sleep—supplemented by catnaps during the day, if you can take some—part of your regular fitness regimen. Your skin (and your waistline) will thank you!

Physical intimacy is another great form of exercise. Sex can directly help your skin by providing a boost to your immune system and an increase in circulation. It helps you to work up a sweat, which lets your body release toxins. Progesterone, a hormone that is produced as a by-product of sexual intimacy, acts as an acne inhibitor. As an added bonus, the unmistakable rosy afterglow looks great on everyone!

The stress-reducing benefits of sex are long-lasting, too. A 2005 study found that people who engaged in intercourse within two weeks prior

ALISA'S BODY SAVER

One of the truly pleasant aspects of exercising is that there are plenty of options. Exercise can be as simple as walking, taking up a recreational sport, participating in an exercise class, or following a workout video at home.

ALISA'S BODY SAVER

If you are having trouble falling asleep, avoid exercising within four hours of going to bed. Instead, try to make exercise one of the first things you do to start your day.

to public speaking or other stressful activity had a much easier time handling anxiety; their blood pressure spiked less and returned to normal levels more quickly than that of subjects who hadn't engaged in intercourse.

For the best results, don't just lie there—get busy and move around. When performed actively, sex trains quite a few major muscle groups. One recent study concluded that couples who enjoy sexual relations two or three times a week look two or three years younger than those who aren't sexually active or aren't experiencing satisfactory physical intimacy. As you age, there's a direct correlation between enjoying a satisfactory sex life and maintaining overall good health. Each contributes to the other.

Making Your Move: Motivating Yourself for Fitness

If you don't have a regular fitness program, or if you've had to let your program lapse as you've dealt with other health challenges, I want to encourage you to make a start—or a fresh start—today. Because it's easy to come up with excuses for shortchanging ourselves, especially in the area of health and fitness, I've asked Alisa to share tips for motivating you. She motivated the *Extreme Makeover* participants, and she does the same for her private clients today. The benefits of these practices far outweigh the extra time they take. Before you know it, you'll be basking in the healthy glow of your reflection as your new level of overall fitness shows on your skin. Here are the tips:

Turn obstacles into opportunities. A small change in daily habits can add up to great health gains. Start by viewing obstacles as opportunities. Instead of circling the parking lot looking for a closer spot, park farther away and walk. Take the stairs whenever you can. Play more outdoor games with the kids and vigorously engage in household chores like vacuuming and gardening. Learn to create small energetic games for yourself. One of my favorites is the "Ten-Minute

Cleanup." I race around the house as fast as I can for ten minutes to see how much I can pick up and put away. Many common daily routines offer an opportunity to fit in extra exercise.

Feel pleasure today. Have fun with fitness. Break out of your comfort zone and try a new activity. Go for a swim at a pool in a local college or recreation center. Play a game of Ping Pong, badminton, or disc golf. Visit a local ice skating rink or tennis court. Take some dancing lessons. Think about all the fun things you have watched others do over the years. Think back to your childhood, when simply rolling downhill was fun. There is nothing stopping you from finding a physical activity that brings you pleasure today. When your physical activity gives you joy, you'll be more likely to continue it.

Make time. Try to approach exercise from a place of honesty. There is a big difference between being physically able to do something and making the time to do it. If you wait until you have the time to take a walk, you may never get going. It's important to remember that you already have the time you need to be active—you just need to look at how you are using that time. Take this opportunity to see how you can rearrange your day to free up time for fitness. In order to achieve maximum results, set realistic short-term and long-term fitness goals—for example, "I will take a brisk walk for at least thirty minutes four days this week."

Set yourself up. Learn to set yourself up for success. Invest in simple exercise items such as resistance bands and a few small hand weights ranging from two to five pounds. Purchase a foam roller to help you stretch out a tight back and other limbs. If your budget allows, invest in a simple treadmill so that you can do cardio on a flexible timetable and when the weather keeps you indoors.

Don't go it alone. You might want to find an exercise buddy. This will keep you accountable and can add a new level of fun to your fitness experience. Purchase a pedometer and keep track of your daily steps. A good goal is to walk five miles a day (approximately ten thousand steps). Get inspired and start a morning walking club, or incorporate exercise as a means of being of service in your local community.

Support your motivation. Before beginning or adding to any fitness program, talk with your health care team or schedule a baseline physical if you're not currently in treatment. Track your progress with an exercise journal. Record your physical activity—in any form—over time. Note the activities that give you the most joy and leave you feeling energized.

Alisa's Fitness Tips

Now that you understand the connection between fitness and healthy skin, Alisa will provide tips for making fitness a part of your life every day, starting today. Atthe end of the chapter you will find an illustrated four-day fitness plan that you can make your own.

Fueling Your Workout

- Muscle needs proper nutrition in order to grow. If you skip meals, your workout efforts will not be maximized and your skin can suffer. To give yourself and your body every advantage, start your fitness engine immediately by eating breakfast every morning.
- Consuming five to seven small snacks and meals a day is a great way to rev up your weight-loss engine and stabilize your blood sugar level.
- For full muscle development, always consume a carbohydrate coupled with protein before and after weight training. This will enable you to pump up your muscles, and over time it will help your skin to look better, too. Some great pre- and postworkout food combinations are yam and lean chicken breast, oatmeal and egg whites, and sweet potato and turkey breast.
- Avoid the trap of consuming sugar-filled sports drinks and calorie-laden fitness water when you exercise. Stay hydrated with actual water. Take a liter bottle with you to the gym. Check the label

carefully for hidden sodium content, artificial sweeteners, and potassium benzoate.

Good Form and Equipment

- When you work out, be mindful of your form and posture. Poor form can result in injury. Keep your abdominal muscles tight and contracted, your knees aligned over your feet, and your buttocks tucked in to engage and align your back properly.
- Adequate footwear is a must! Wear shoes that match your activity, foot structure, and lifestyle. Always replace footwear before it wears out. A pair of shoes may still look good, but studies show that with frequent use, fitness shoes can lose one-third of their shock-absorbing ability in a matter of months. Find an athletic footwear store that will help you to choose shoes that are customized to you and your needs, not based on what they have in stock.
- Your muscles actively take shape as they contract. The more time you spend squeezing your muscles, the tighter your body will become. Practice squeezing your butt and other muscle groups as you go about your day. Over time this activity will tone, tighten, and firm your body.
- Stretching for five to ten minutes after every workout will improve recovery time and prevent injury. Stretching benefits your body and the overall appearance of your skin.

Proper Weight Training

- Incorporate weight training into your life with a one-hour session three or four times a week. Start slowly and seek guidance from a knowledgeable personal trainer.
- Focus on muscle contraction, and be sure to control your movement. Jerking movements and flailing limbs can overstress joints and set the stage for injury.
- Actively squeeze your muscles and keep them contracted as you move through your weight-training routine.

- When you weight-train, try placing one hand on the muscle you are training. This should help you to focus on contraction and increase the effectiveness of your workout. If you feel tension growing in your neck, stop the exercise and take a few slow, deep breaths. Lifting your chin when you resume the exercise will also help you to release tension. The goal is to feel a contraction only in the muscle that you are trying to work, not anywhere else.
- Develop a schedule that alternates different body parts throughout the week.

The Importance of Rest

- Rest your body, and your shape will change.
- Overexertion and pushing yourself too hard can place your body in a state of distress. Overtraining and not getting enough sleep will inhibit your body's repair cycle, including the repair of your skin.
- Allow a minimum of seventy-two hours of rest before resistance training the same muscle group again.
- Stay calm to make the most of your fitness routine. Stress in any form—from work, traffic, or even overtraining—will have a major impact on your progress. Your body interprets all forms of stress as a signal to protect itself, which means that it will hold onto its fat reserves however it can.
- If you are feeling tired, listen to your body and take the day off from exercise.

Joining a Gym

If gyms make you nervous because you think you don't "belong" there, I'm here to tell you that you belong anywhere you'd like to go. It doesn't matter how old, inexperienced, heavy, or out of shape you think you might be; gyms are for people who want to improve their health. All you need is a simple desire to walk through the front door. If you do not have a gym membership, here are some key points to consider:

- The gym must be convenient. It should be close to either your home or your workplace. If the gym is not conveniently located, you will end up going infrequently, if at all.

- Obtain a guest pass and try out the gym before you join. See if the environment suits your personality. Some people enjoy the energy of muscle-bound individuals pumping weights. Others prefer a more serene atmosphere. You can also buddy up and find a friend to go to the gym with you.

- Gyms are for everyone, not just for people who are fit and skinny. It is completely normal to feel out of place in a new gym. That feeling will go away the more you visit the gym and go about your workout.

- If you don't know how a piece of equipment works, don't be afraid to ask someone at the front desk. You might feel silly, but don't worry—people ask these questions all day, every day. It's important for you to know how to operate gym equipment safely and effectively.

Finally, remember that the process of attaining a healthy body and beautiful skin begins in the mind. When embarking on a fitness lifestyle change, set yourself up to succeed by starting with a positive attitude. When you adopt a positive mind-set, you increase your chances of success and empower those around you. Learn to approach your new exercise habits with joy, and your rate of physical success will skyrocket.

Alisa's Four-Day-a-Week Fitness Plan

Practice the following four-day routine to immediately jump-start your fitness level, increase your vitality, and bring your body and spirit into balance.

Unless otherwise noted, perform each exercise until you feel a burn, and then do three or four more repetitions beyond that point.

Day 1

1. Perform 30 to 45 minutes of cardio on a treadmill.
2. Do 5 to 10 minutes of stretching (see the stretches at the end of this chapter).
3. Train your legs for 20 minutes. Do 2 or 3 sets of each of the leg exercises described below, depending on your fitness level. Remember to rest for 2 minutes between each set.
4. Perform 2 or 3 sets of low abdominal breathing exercises (see the instructions at the end of this chapter).
5. Perform the three yoga poses.

LEG EXERCISES

Short-Range Standing Squats

Starting Position
- Start by holding onto something sturdy that does not move and that will support your weight.
- Place your feet slightly wider than shoulder-width apart, with your toes pointing forty-five degrees away from the center.
- Inhale deeply and begin to exhale as you start the movement.

Movement
- Slowly exhale and lower yourself slowly so that you are slightly bending your knees, about halfway to a sitting position.
- Squeeze your gluteal muscles and tighten your inner thighs.
- Slowly raise yourself to the starting position while exhaling completely.
- Slowly repeat this exercise thirteen to eighteen times.

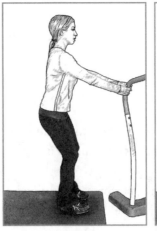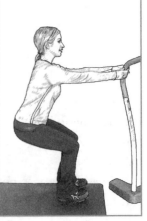

Hip Abductor, Toes Out

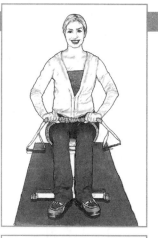

Starting Position

- Sit comfortably in a chair with back support and with a height that allows you to keep your feet planted flat on the floor.
- Wrap an exercise band around your thighs just above knee level.
- Your knees should be shoulder-width apart, with your heels touching each other and your toes forty-five degrees away from each other.
- Inhale deeply and begin to exhale as you start the movement.

Movement

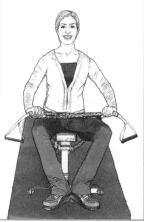

- Keep the band at the same tension throughout the entire movement.
- Slowly exhale and focus your attention on the outer thighs as you slowly separate your legs as far as is comfortable.
- Hold the contraction for 2 or 3 seconds.
- Slowly return your legs to the starting position while exhaling completely.
- Slowly repeat this exercise thirteen to eighteen times.

Hip Abductor, Heels Out

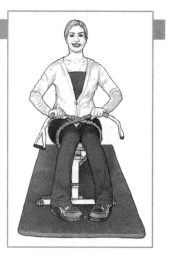

Starting Position

- Sit comfortably in a chair with back support and with a height that allows you to keep your feet planted flat on the floor.
- Lean forward slightly and wrap an exercise band around your thighs just above the knees.
- Your knees should be shoulder-width apart, with your toes pointed in toward each other and your heels out.
- Inhale deeply and begin to exhale as you start the movement.

Movement

- Lean slightly forward and maintain constant tension in the exercise band. Slowly exhale and move your legs apart from each other while keeping your feet in the same place.
- Consciously focus on the upper part of the gluteal muscles right below the back.
- Hold the contraction for 3 to 5 seconds.
- Slowly return to the starting position while finishing your exhalation.
- Slowly repeat this exercise thirteen to eighteen times.

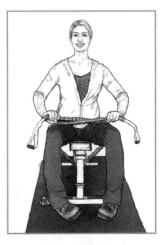

Wall Squats

Starting Position

- Start with your back pressed firmly against a wall or a doorjamb (but not a mirror or any other glass surface).
- Keep your feet planted firmly on the floor about shoulder-width apart and facing straight ahead.
- To prevent knee injury, your feet should be far enough away from the wall/doorjamb so that your knees do *not* extend past your feet as you squat down.
- Inhale deeply and begin to exhale as you start the movement.

Movement

- Slowly exhale and lower yourself so that your knees are bent at a ninety-degree angle.
- Squeeze your thigh and gluteal muscles and hold the contraction for one or two seconds.
- Slowly raise yourself back to the starting position as you complete your exhale. Slowly repeat this exercise thirteen to eighteen times.

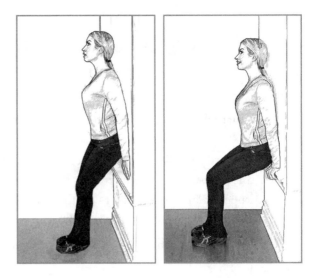

Full-Range Leg Extensions

Starting Position

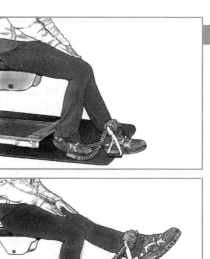

- Sit in a chair with back support and hold onto the side of the chair for stability.
- During the initial contractions you will want to place your hands on your thigh muscles for a moment to feel the strength of the contraction.
- Start with your knees bent at a ninety-degree angle.
- Tie an exercise band in a ring, then step on the band with one foot and attach it to the other ankle to perform the exercise one leg at a time for better concentration. (Alternately, you can wrap the exercise band around your toes and attach it to the chair legs.)
- Inhale deeply and begin to exhale as you start the movement.

Movement

- Point your toes like a ballerina and extend your thigh in a controlled movement so that your legs are straight out in front of you.
- Slowly lower your legs to the starting position.
- Do not hold the contraction for this exercise.
- Slowly repeat this exercise thirteen to eighteen times.

Full-Range Hamstring Curl

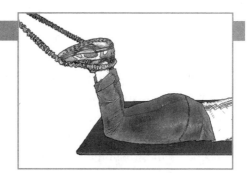

Starting Position

- Lie on your stomach with an exercise band wrapped around your ankles and attached to something that doesn't move.
- Inhale deeply and begin to exhale as you start the movement.

Movement

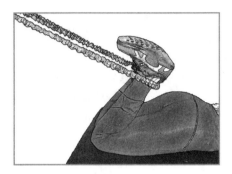

- Slowly exhale as you curl your feet back toward your gluteal muscles while keeping your toes flexed up toward your knees.
- Hold the contraction for 3 to 5 seconds.
- Slowly lower your legs back to the starting position as you complete your exhalation.
- Slowly repeat this exercise thirteen to eighteen times.

YOGA POSES

Child Pose

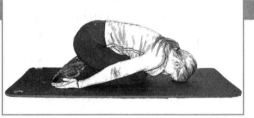

- Start this pose on your hands and knees with your toes outstretched behind you.
- Rock backward so that your gluteal muscles are resting on your heels.
- Slowly lower your forehead to the floor and move your arms to your sides, stretched out behind you with your palms up.
- Rest the tops of your hands on the floor and hold this pose for a few seconds. You may also perform the child pose between other poses to rest.

Cobra Pose

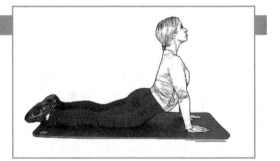

- Lie flat on the floor. Draw your legs back while keeping the tops of your feet on the floor. Stretch your hands on the floor under your shoulders. Hold your elbows close to your body.
- Press the tops of your thighs, feet, and pubic bone strongly into the floor.
- Breathe in and straighten the arms to elevate your chest off the floor.

Compress your tailbone toward your pubic bone and elevate the pubic bone toward the belly button. Taper the hip points. Your buttocks should remain lightly firm.

- Tighten both your shoulder blades against your back. Expand your side ribs forward. Elevate through the top of the sternum but do not push the front ribs forward. Make sure your back bends evenly throughout your spine.
- Hold this pose for 30 seconds, making sure you can breathe easily. Finish by exhaling and releasing the pose.

Plank Pose

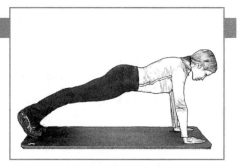

- Start this pose on your hands and knees with your palms flat on the floor, your fingers pointed in the direction that your head is pointed, and your shoulders fully extended.
- One leg at a time, straighten each leg so that you are resting on your toes.
- Keep your back perfectly straight like a plank and hold that position for 10 seconds.
- Do not move, and do not let your back start to arch or droop.
- This is similar to what a push-up looks like, except that you do not press up and down—you simply hold the position.

Day 2

1. Perform 30 to 45 minutes of cardio on a treadmill.
2. Do 5 to 10 minutes of stretching (see the stretches at the end of this chapter).
3. Train your shoulders for 30 minutes. Do 2 or 3 sets of each exercise described below, depending on your fitness level. Remember to rest for 2 minutes between each set.
4. Perform 2 or 3 sets of low abdominal breathing exercises (see the instructions at the end of this chapter).
5. Perform the two yoga poses.

SHOULDER EXERCISES

External Rotator Cuff, Part 1

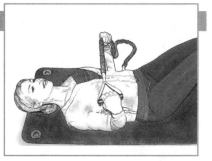

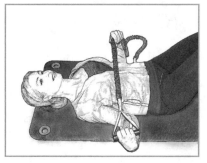

Starting Position

- Begin on your back, holding the handle of an exercise band with one hand and the midpoint of the band with the other hand. (Do not use dumbbells for this exercise—they aren't effective.)
- Place your elbow (on the side holding the handle) as close to your rib cage as possible. Do not move it away from your rib cage during the exercise.
- You should maintain a ninety-degree angle at your elbow and keep your wrists turned in.

Movement

- While keeping your wrists turned in, rotate your arm (on the side holding the handle) out as if the shoulder were a hinge.
- Do not move your elbow away from your rib cage.
- You should rotate out only as far as you can without moving your entire arm.
- Hold the contraction for a couple of seconds.
- Breathe in as you return to the starting position.
- Slowly repeat this exercise thirteen to eighteen times.
- Perform the same steps with the opposite arm, or you can alternate hands.

External Rotator Cuff, Part 2

Starting Position

- Start on your back, with an exercise band hooked around your feet or another stable object and the handles in your hands.
- Raise your arms over your head so that you have a ninety-degree angle at your underarms and a ninety-degree angle at your elbows.

- Start with your forearms at ninety-degree angles to the floor.

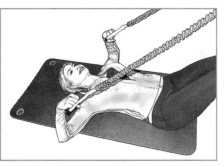

Movement

- Without moving your elbows at all, rotate your shoulders slowly so that your forearms rotate as far back as is comfortably possible. Ultimately, you want your forearms to be parallel to the floor.
- You do not have to rotate completely.
- Rotate only until you are comfortable without arching your back.
- Hold the contraction for a split second.
- Slowly return your arms to the starting position.
- Slowly repeat this exercise thirteen to eighteen times.

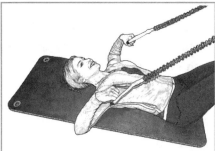

Posterior Deltoid Fly

Starting Position

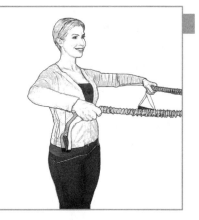

- Stand (alternately you can perform this sitting in a chair with back support) with an exercise band attached to something stable that does not move.
- Hold the exercise band slightly ahead of the handles so that your palms face the floor and your thumbs wrap completely around the band.
- Relax your shoulders by shaking them out a bit.
- Keep your elbows slightly bent.
- Take a big inhalation, and as you begin the motion, exhale through the movement.

Movement

- Without using the muscles in the middle of your back or neck, slowly pull your arms away from each other while maintaining your wrist and elbow positions exactly.
- Focus on the muscles in the back of the shoulders as you breathe out through the movement.
- When your hands are in line across your shoulders, pause for a split second and slowly return them to the starting position.
- Repeat this exercise thirteen to eighteen times.

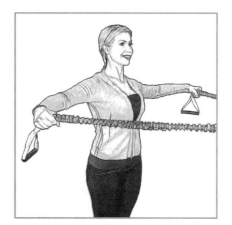

Front Deltoid Raise

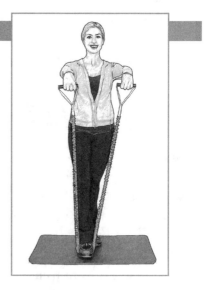

Starting Position

- Stand with your feet together and with a slight bend at the knees.
- Keep your body relaxed, especially your neck and wrists.
- Hold an exercise band or a dumbbell with your palms down, your wrists slightly bent down, and your elbows pointing out away from each other.
- Take a big breath in, and as you begin the movement, slowly start to breathe out.

Movement

- Raise your arms directly in front of you in unison to just above parallel.
- Make sure that your elbows stay slightly bent and are facing away from each other.
- Breathe in as you return to the starting position.
- Slowly repeat this exercise thirteen to eighteen times.

Short-Range Lateral Deltoid Raise

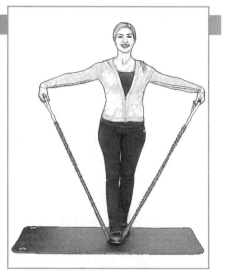

Starting Position

- Start with your feet together, your knees slightly bent, and your arms at your sides.
- Relax your whole body, especially your neck.
- Hold an exercise band or a dumbbell in your hands with your palms facing the floor.
- Bend your wrists down toward the forearms.
- Bend your elbows slightly so that they bow away from your torso.
- Inhale deeply, and as you begin to raise your arms, slowly exhale.

Movement

- Slowly raise your arms out to the side, leading with your elbows and keeping your wrists limp.
- Do not allow your shoulders to scrunch up. If necessary, limit the range of motion to about two-thirds of the way up.
- Hold the contraction until you exhale fully.
- Inhale as you lower your arms back to the starting position.
- Slowly repeat this exercise thirteen to eighteen times.

YOGA POSES

Cat Cow Pose

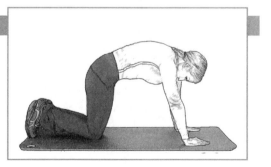

- For the cow part of the pose, start on your hands and knees with your back in a straight line and your palms flat on the floor, your fingers pointing forward.
- Relax your feet so that the tops of your feet lie flat on the ground with your toes curled slightly.
- Take a big inhalation and drop your belly toward the floor while simultaneously shifting your head and face toward the ceiling.

- Envision your back as a perfect arc from the tailbone to the top of your spine.
- Move into the cat part of the pose. As you exhale, slowly and deliberately arch your spine in the other direction so that your head is down and your back is arched up toward the ceiling, like a black cat on Halloween.
- Make sure that your breathing matches the movement in your spine, and repeat the pose for 5 to 8 breaths.

Camel Pose

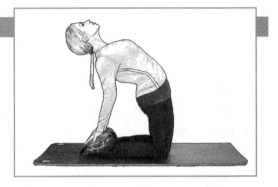

- Start by kneeling on the floor with your knees hip-width apart and your thighs at a ninety-degree angle to the ground. Narrow both hip points, firm your buttocks, and rotate your thighs slightly inward. Relax your outer hips and keep them soft. Press the tops of your feet as well as your shins directly into the floor.
- Relax your hands on the back of your pelvis. The bases of both palms should lie on the tops of the buttocks, with all fingers pointing downward. Use your hands to spread the back pelvis and lengthen it down through your tailbone. Gently firm the rear forward, in the direction of the pubic bone. Take a deep breath in and elevate your heart by pushing both shoulder blades against the back ribs.
- Recline backward against the hardness of the tailbone and both shoulder blades. Keep your head up, your hands on your pelvis, and your chin tucked into your sternum in the initial stages of this pose.

    (If you are new to yoga or are very tight, you probably want to ease into this pose. In that case, keep your pelvis at a slight angle and walk one hand back toward your foot slowly. Then press your hips forward so that your pelvis is at a right angle to the floor and touch your other hand to the foot on that side. Ideally, you want to touch your hands to your feet while keeping your thighs at right angles to the floor. If you are unable to touch your feet without putting undue pressure on your lower back, position your toes under and lift your heels.)

- Make sure that your ribs are not exaggeratedly extended toward the sky, which will arch your back and compress your vertebrae. Tilt your pelvis up toward your rib cage while releasing your front ribs. Now lift your lower-back ribs away from your pelvis to keep your lower vertebrae fully lengthened.
- Press your hands against the soles or heels of your feet with your fingers pointing down toward the floor. Turn your elbows forward while keeping your shoulder blades relaxed. Keep your neck relaxed or slightly tilted back. Make sure that it is not tensed.
- Maintain the pose for 30 seconds.
- Come out of the pose slowly by bringing your hands to your hips. Take a deep breath in and lift your head and torso up by pushing your hips toward the floor. Always come out of this pose chest first; do not lead with your head when exiting this pose.

Day 3

1. Perform 30 to 45 minutes of cardio on a treadmill.
2. Do 5 to 10 minutes of stretching (see the stretches at the end of this chapter).
3. Train your biceps for 10 minutes. Do 2 or 3 sets of the exercise described below, depending on your fitness level. Remember to rest for 2 minutes between each set.
4. Train your back for 20 minutes. Do 2 or 3 sets of the exercises described below, depending on your fitness level. Remember to rest for 2 minutes between each set.
5. Perform two or three sets of low abdominal breathing exercises (see the instructions at the end of this chapter).
6. Perform the two yoga poses.

BICEPS EXERCISES

Short-Range Biceps Curl

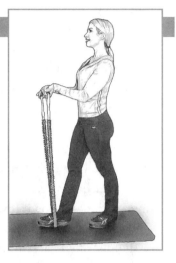

Starting Position
- Keep your feet slightly apart and your knees slightly bent.
- Start with your arms at your sides while holding an exercise band or dumbbells.
- Place your elbows slightly in front of your rib cage and bend them slightly.
- Inhale deeply as you relax your entire body, and as you are beginning the motion, slowly start to exhale.

Movement
- Slowly squeeze your biceps (the muscles in the front of the upper arms) as you exhale, and begin raising your arms in unison.
- Curl your arms halfway up while squeezing the biceps.
- Breathe in as you return to the starting position.
- Slowly repeat this exercise thirteen to eighteen times.
- You should perform the exercise until you feel a burn and then do 3 or 4 more repetitions.

BACK EXERCISES

Wide-Grip Pull-Down

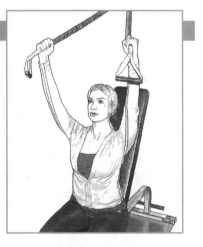

Starting Position
- Sit in a chair with back support.
- Attach an exercise band to something sturdy that does not move and that is above your head, such as a doorjamb.
- Hold the exercise band above the handle so that your thumbs completely wrap around.
- Place your elbows slightly in front of your face.

- Take a big inhalation, and as you begin the movement, slowly exhale.

Movement

- Lower your arms about halfway so that you feel the contraction right under the armpits.
- Breathe in as you return to the starting position.
- Slowly repeat this exercise thirteen to eighteen times.

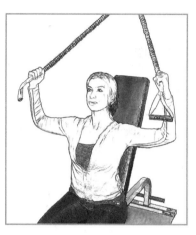

High-Seated Row

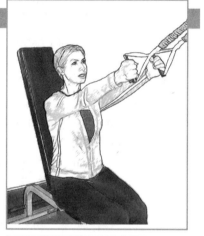

Starting Position

- Sit in a chair, but not all the way back to the backrest, so that your elbows can move in a linear path.
- Attach an exercise band to something stable that does not move and that is slightly higher than your head.
- Sit up straight and tilt your chin up at a forty-five-degree angle.
- Relax your shoulder and neck muscles and inhale deeply.
- Slowly exhale as you begin the motion.

Movement

- Squeeze the muscles between your shoulder blades as you pull your arms backward.
- Pull your arms all the way back as you visualize your elbows coming together behind your back.
- Hold the contraction for 2 seconds.
- Breathe in as you return to the starting position.
- Slowly repeat this exercise thirteen to eighteen times.

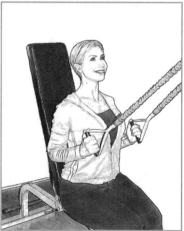

YOGA POSES

Lion Pose

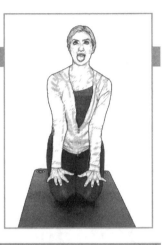

- Cross the front of your right ankle over the back of your left ankle while kneeling on the floor. Both feet will point out on either side. Sit back onto the top of your right heel.
- With your palms pressed firmly against your knees, exhale loudly and forcefully while fanning the palms and splaying your fingers like a lion's claws.

Downward-Facing Dog

- Start this pose on your hands and knees with your palms flat on the floor, your fingers pointed straight ahead, and your shoulders fully extended.
- While keeping your back perfectly flat, take your knees off the floor and lift your gluteal muscles straight into the air.
- Keep your feet flat on the ground, straighten your knees, and lift your gluteal muscles up high.

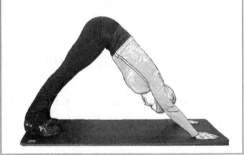

- Your stance should be that of a pyramid, with your gluteal muscles at the apex.

Day 4

1. Perform 30 to 45 minutes of cardio on a treadmill.
2. Do 5 to 10 minutes of stretching (see the stretches at the end of this chapter).
3. Train your chest for 20 to 30 minutes. Do 2 or 3 sets of the exercises described below, depending on your fitness level. Remember to rest for 2 minutes between each set.
4. Train your triceps (the muscles in the back of the upper arms) for

10 to 15 minutes. Do 2 or 3 sets of the exercise described below, depending on your fitness level. Remember to rest for 2 minutes between each set.

5. Perform two or three sets of low abdominal breathing exercises (see the instructions at the end of this chapter).

6. Perform the two yoga poses.

CHEST EXERCISES

Full-Range Chest Fly

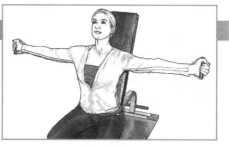

Starting Position

- Sit in a chair with back support.
- Attach an exercise band to something low that is sturdy and that does not move.
- Keep your elbows up and out, and do not let them drop to your sides at any time during the exercise.
- Take a big inhalation, and as you begin the movement, slowly exhale.

Movement

- Using your upper chest and not your shoulders, slowly and deliberately push the handles away from you while maintaining your elbow height.
- Do not fully extend your arms so that your elbows are straight.
- Instead, stop the range of motion while there is still a slight bend in your elbows.
- Breathe in as you return to the starting position.
- Slowly repeat this exercise thirteen to eighteen times.

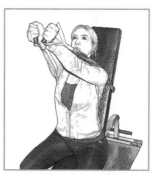

Short-Range Chest Fly

Starting Position

- Sit in a chair with back support.
- Attach an exercise band to something directly behind you that is sturdy and that does not move.

- Keep your elbows up and out, and do not let them drop to your sides at any time during the exercise.
- Take a big inhalation, and as you begin the movement, slowly exhale.

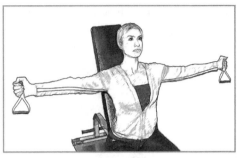

Movement

- Using the edge of your chest and not your shoulders or arms, slowly and deliberately pull the band forward about 4 inches.
- Do not follow the range of motion all the way to the center of your chest. This exercise is only for the edge of the chest, to lift and provide definition.
- Breathe in as you return to the starting position.
- Slowly repeat this exercise thirteen to eighteen times.

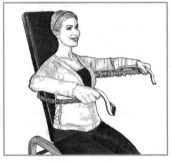

TRICEPS EXERCISE

Reverse-Grip Triceps Pull-Down

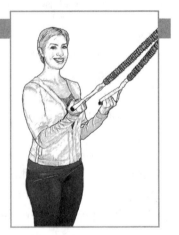

Starting Position

- Stand with your posture as straight as is comfortable. (Alternately, you can sit in a chair with back support.)
- Attach an exercise band to something sturdy that does not move and that is higher than your head.
- Pin your elbows to your sides and make sure that your arms do not swing during the exercise.
- Hold the handles of the band with your palms facing you and your elbows bent.
- Take a big inhalation, and as you begin the movement, slowly exhale.

Movement

- Keeping your wrists pivoted so that your pinky fingers are next to your body, and without moving your elbows at all, extend your arms all the way back.

- Consciously squeeze the backs of your arms and hold the contraction for 3 to 5 seconds.
- Force your knuckles to come back slightly, as though they were trying to touch the tops of your forearms.
- Breathe in as you return to the starting position.
- Slowly repeat this exercise thirteen to eighteen times.

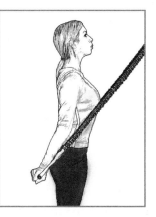

YOGA POSES

Forward Elbow Clasp

- Stand with both arms placed at your sides and your feet at hip-width apart.
- Keep a flat back and both feet grounded as you fold forward from your hips.
- Proceed until your torso is draping from your hips.
- Grasp each of your elbows with the opposite hand. While keeping your legs firm, allow your torso to flow out of your waist.
- Hold this position for 3 to 10 breaths.
- Gradually elevate your abdominal muscles toward your spine as you release the position. Remember to keep a flat back as you bring your body to an erect position. Finally, disengage your elbows.

Face Massage

- Sit in a comfortable place on the floor.
- With your eyes closed, rub your hands together rapidly until they are warm.
- Place your fingertips on your eyebrows, with your little fingers next to each other. Press firmly along your brows and simultaneously trace each brow with its hand until your hands reach your temples.
- Duplicate this motion multiple times. With every repetition, move up a quarter inch until you've reached your hairline.

- Next, position the tips of your fingers on the bridge of your nose. In one downward motion, swipe your fingertips along your cheek-bones.

For Any Day of the Week

Deep Breathing

Once you have mastered this technique, you can practice deep breathing in any position, even while driving your car or working at your computer.

Low Abdominal Breathing

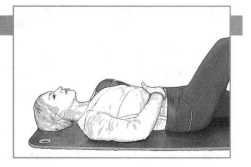

Starting Position
- Lie on your back with your knees bent and your feet flat on the floor.
- Take a big inhalation and fill your diaphragm with air.
- Start to exhale as you begin the exercise.

Exercise
- Breathe all the air out of your lungs and belly.
- Pull your belly button toward your spine.
- Cramp the abdominal muscles so that your pelvis tilts slightly upward.
- Hold the contraction for 1 to 5 seconds (depending on your fitness level).
- Relax your abdominal muscles and begin to inhale again.
- Repeat the exercise twenty to twenty-five times, slowly and without hyperventilating.

Stretching

Do 5 to 10 minutes of stretching before exercising and another 5 to 10 minutes after you are finished with your workout.

Hamstring Stretch

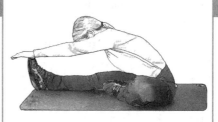

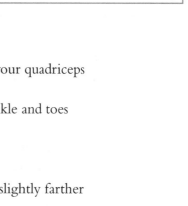

Starting Position

- Sit with your left leg extended in front of you and your toes pointed up toward the ceiling.
- Bend your right leg so that your right foot touches the inside of your left knee.

Stretch

- Place your right hand over your left hand.
- Extend your hands toward your left toes while flexing your quadriceps (upper thigh).
- Keep your lower back perfectly straight and your left ankle and toes relaxed.
- Stretch only as far as is comfortable.
- Hold the stretch for 10 seconds, then relax.
- Repeat the process four to six times, trying to stretch slightly farther each time.
- Repeat with the right leg.

Calf Stretch

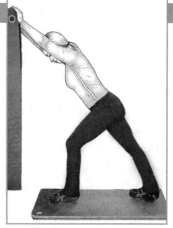

Starting Position

- Stand about 1 foot away from a wall, with your arms outstretched toward the wall.
- Bend your arms at the elbows and place your forearms against the wall.

Stretch

- Keep your right foot flat on the floor and slightly bend both knees.
- Place the ball of your left foot against the wall and lean into the wall until you feel the stretch in your right calf muscle while also pulling up with your shin muscle.
- Stretch only as far as is comfortable.
- Hold the stretch for 10 seconds, then relax.

- Repeat the process four to six times, trying to stretch slightly farther each time.
- Repeat with the left calf muscle.

Quadriceps Stretch

Starting Position
- Support yourself with your left arm against a wall or a sturdy object.
- Bend your left leg behind you so that you can hold your ankle with your right hand.
- Make sure that you are stable and not wobbly or unbalanced.

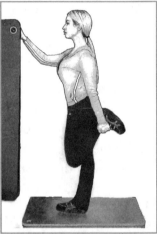

Stretch
- Pull your left leg with your right hand until your heel touches your gluteal muscles or until you feel a stretch in the thigh muscles.
- Stretch only as far as is comfortable.
- Hold the stretch for 10 seconds, then relax.
- Repeat the process four to six times, trying to stretch slightly farther each time.
- Repeat with the right leg.

Inner Thigh Stretch

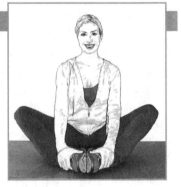

Starting Position
- Sit on the floor with your back supported against a wall or another secure object.
- Pull both feet toward each other in front of you and sit cross-legged, "Indian style."
- Hold both feet with your hands and rest your elbows on your legs.

Stretch
- Press down on your legs slightly with your elbows.
- At the same time, pull your legs toward the floor and lean slightly into the stretch.

- Stretch only as far as is comfortable.
- Hold the stretch for 10 seconds, then relax.
- Repeat the process four to six times, trying to stretch slightly farther each time.

Triceps Stretch

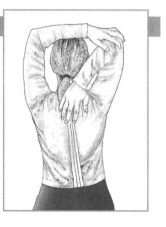

Starting Position
- Stand with your back straight and your body relaxed.
- Bend your left arm over your head so that your palm rests on the upper middle part of your back, your fingers facing the floor.

Stretch
- Use your left hand to push your right elbow down slightly so that your right hand moves farther down your back.
- Stretch only as far as is comfortable.
- Hold the stretch for 10 seconds, then relax.
- Repeat the process four to six times, trying to stretch slightly farther each time.
- Repeat with the right arm.

Shoulder Stretch

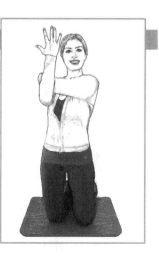

Starting Position
- Stretch your left arm out in front of you with your palm facing the floor.
- Place the palm of your right hand on your left triceps.

Stretch
- Using only slight pressure, pull your left arm across your body with your right arm.
- Stretch only as far as is comfortable.
- Hold the stretch for 10 seconds, then relax.
- Repeat the process four to six times, trying to stretch slightly farther each time.
- Repeat with the right arm.

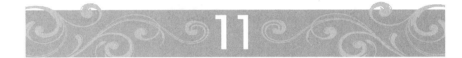

At-Home Skin Care Recipes

Homemade skin care products are a great way to nourish your skin and are fun and easy to make. When you make your own skin care products, you know what each contains, can avoid harmful ingredients, and select ones that are right for your individual skin needs. The following recipes were formulated using the most up-to-date information and will remedy the skin conditions discussed in this book. Making them is much like following a cookbook. I had a great time making them in the kitchen and testing them on my own skin!

Some Recipe Guidelines

- When milk—either liquid or powdered—is called for in the recipes, always use whole, not low-fat or nonfat. Yogurt should also be whole and plain.
- For recipes that call for a base cream or a lotion, use CeraVe, Vani-cream, or a basic cold cream with no added ingredients. The cream

should be at room temperature when you mix in the other ingredients.

- Always use glass bowls and jars to mix and to store homemade products. Glass is not only safe to sterilize, but it will not react with the naturally occurring acids present in many of these fresh ingredients. To sterilize, soak your glassware in very hot water mixed with soap and one tablespoon of bleach for about fifteen minutes. Then rinse under hot water to remove the soap and bleach. Wipe dry. Make sure to store any remaining homemade skin care products in a sealed jar.
- All fruits and vegetables should be fresh unless otherwise noted.
- Each recipe is coded for various skin types and problems, as shown in the chart below.

DR. AVA'S SKIN-ISSUE GRID

ACNE		PREGNANCY		MENOPAUSE		CHEMOTHERAPY		POST CHEMOTHERAPY	
A	all skin types	P	all skin types	M	all skin types	C	all skin types	PCA	all skin types
AO	oily skin	PO	oily skin	MO	oily skin	CO	oily skin	PCO	oily skin
AC	combination skin	PC	combination skin	MC	combination skin	CC	combination skin	PCC	combination skin
AD	dry skin	PD	dry skin	MD	dry skin	CD	dry skin	PCD	dry skin

Cleansers

PAPAYA-LEMON CLEANSER

½ papaya
2 tablespoons witch hazel

1 teaspoon lemon juice

AO, AC, PO, MO, MC, CO, PCO, PCC

Peel and dice papaya (no seeds) and blend with witch hazel. Add lemon juice, and blend again briefly. Use warm water to moisten a washcloth. Add 2 tablespoons of the cleanser to the washcloth and gently rub your face to cleanse. Rinse off with warm water. Store the cleanser in a sealed jar.

GRAPE AND HONEY
CLEANSER

AC, AD, PC, PD,
MC, MD, CC,
CD, PCC, PCD

1 cup grapes with seeds
1 teaspoon honey
1 teaspoon olive oil

½ teaspoon baking soda
5 tablespoons milk

Use a blender to mix grapes, honey, and olive oil. (Make sure the grapes are well mashed.) Add baking soda and milk. Blend on a slow speed until mixed well. Refrigerate the cleanser in a sealed jar. Wash your face with the cleanser in the morning and/or the evening.

STRAWBERRY AND HONEY
CLEANSER

AO, AC, MO,
PCO

3 or 4 very ripe strawberries, hulled
½ teaspoon honey

2 drops lavender oil

Crush strawberries through a sieve, retaining the juice in a small glass bowl. Add honey and lavender oil to the strawberry juice and mix well. Massage the mixture firmly onto your face and your neck. Leave on for one minute, then rinse off with warm water.

MILKY CLEANSER

AD, PD, MD,
CD, PCD

2 tablespoons milk or cream
1 tablespoon almond oil

2 teaspoons almond meal
1 teaspoon honey

Mix all ingredients in a glass dish. Dampen your face and dip a cotton pad in the cleanser. Gently wipe your face, then rinse off with warm water.

LEMON CLEANSER

AO, MO, PO,
PCO

¼ cup witch hazel
1 teaspoon baking soda

1 teaspoon lemon juice

Combine all ingredients in a jar. Place a small amount of cleanser on a washcloth and gently wash your face. Rinse off with warm water.

YOGURT CLEANSER

2 tablespoons yogurt   1 tablespoon applesauce
1 teaspoon baking soda

AO, AC, MO, MC, PO, CO, PCO, PCC

Mix all ingredients by hand or in a blender. Using your fingers, gently massage a small amount onto your dampened face. Rinse off with warm water.

GRAPE CLEANSER

15 dark grapes with seeds   1 tablespoon fine cornmeal
1 teaspoon olive oil

A, P, M, PCA

Use a blender to mix grapes (with skin and seeds) and olive oil. Pour into a glass bowl and add cornmeal. Stir until all ingredients are well combined. Pour a small amount onto a wet washcloth and gently cleanse your face. Rinse off with warm water.

EGG WHITE CLEANSER

1 egg white   1 teaspoon baking soda
2 tablespoons yogurt

AO, MO, MC, PO, PC, PCO, PCC

Whisk egg white in a glass bowl until frothy. In a separate bowl, mix yogurt and baking soda, then add egg white. Gently wash your face with the cleanser. Rinse off with warm water.

CALENDULA CLEANSER

2 tablespoons oats   2 teaspoons milk
1 teaspoon calendula extract ½ teaspoon honey

AD, AC, PC, PD, M, C, PCA

Use a blender to grind the oats. Put other ingredients in the blender and combine until creamy. Massage a small amount onto your damp face, neck, and/or chest. Rinse off with warm water.

BAKING SODA CLEANSER

1 teaspoon baking soda   ⅓ cup milk
½ teaspoon honey

A, P, M, PCA

Mix all ingredients in a small glass bowl. Dampen your face and dip gauze into the cleanser. Gently wipe your face and rinse off with warm water.

Mists and Toners

POMEGRANATE-MINT MIST

A, P, M, C, PCA

1 cup water

4 mint leaves, crushed

2 pomegranate tea bags

Boil water. Add mint leaves and pomegranate tea bags. Steep for fifteen minutes. Remove the leaves and bags. Pour the liquid into a jar, seal, and refrigerate. When the liquid is cold, pour some into a small spray bottle. Keep the rest refrigerated.

GREEN TEA–ROSEWATER MIST

A, P, M, C, PCA

½ cup water

2 green tea bags

½ cup rosewater

Boil water, add tea bags, and let steep for 15 minutes. Remove the tea bags and add rosewater. Mix well. Pour into a spray bottle. Refrigerate the rest in a sealed jar.

CHAMOMILE MIST

A, P, M, C, PCA

¼ cup chamomile water

2 tablespoons rose water

Combine ingredients in a bottle. Shake well. Mist your face after cleansing or if your skin feels dehydrated during the day.

CUCUMBER WITH GREEN TEA TONER

A, P, M, C, PCA

¼ cup distilled water

1 green tea bag

1 cucumber

Boil water and brew tea bag. Peel, seed, and cut cucumber into small cubes. Mix cucumber and tea in a blender until you have a thick pulp. Strain through a sieve into a glass bowl. Use a cotton pad or gauze to apply juice to your face, neck, and chest. (Always wash and pat dry those areas first.) You can refrigerate the rest of the product in a jar for up to four days.

SOOTHING GREEN TONER

1 cucumber
½ cup witch hazel
1 cup distilled or pure spring water

2 tablespoons green tea leaves
or 3 green tea bags

A, P, M, C, PCA

Peel cucumber and use a blender to make a puree. Strain the puree through a very fine sieve into a glass bowl and mix juice with witch hazel and water. Boil water and brew green tea leaves (or tea bags). Remove the tea leaves (or bags). Let tea cool before adding it to the juice mixture. Store in the refrigerator.

CITRUS TONER

1 tablespoon lemon juice
1 tablespoon witch hazel

2 tablespoons rosewater

AO, AC, PO, MO, MC, PCO, PCC

Mix all ingredients and store in the refrigerator.

POMEGRANATE TONER

2 tablespoons pomegranate juice
1 tablespoon witch hazel

2 teaspoons vodka
½ teaspoon sea salt

AO, MO, PCO

Combine all ingredients in a bottle. Shake well for a minute. Use a cotton pad or ball to apply to your face. Use every other day, once a day.

HERBAL FACIAL TONER-MIST

⅓ cup distilled water
2 chamomile tea bags
½ teaspoon rosemary extract

½ teaspoon calendula extract
½ cup rosewater

AC, AD, PC, PD, MC, MD, CC, CD, PCC, PCD

Boil water and add chamomile tea bags. Brew for ten minutes, then remove bags and let cool. Combine all ingredients in a jar and shake well. You may mist or wipe your face with this toner.

APPLE TONER-MIST

AO, PO, MO,
CO, PCO

2 tablespoons unsweetened apple juice 1 teaspoon lemon balm water
1 tablespoon witch hazel

Combine all ingredients in a bottle. Shake well. Using cotton pads, gently wipe your face.

Scrubs

SUGAR-APPLE SCRUB

This natural exfoliant is gentle enough to use up to three times a week on acne-prone skin. Green tea has antioxidant properties as well.

AO, AC, PO, PC,
MO, MC, CO,
CC, PCO, PCC

½ cup applesauce, preferably organic   2 tablespoons green tea leaves
  or homemade   2 tablespoons olive oil
3 tablespoons brown sugar

Mix all ingredients in a bowl into a light fluffy paste. Massage onto your clean wet face and rinse off with room-temperature water.

SWEET PINEAPPLE SCRUB

AO, MO

⅓ cup pineapple   2 tablespoons cornmeal
1 teaspoon lemon juice

In a blender, puree pineapple and lemon juice. Mix puree with cornmeal in a glass bowl. Gently massage the mixture onto your clean face for a few minutes, then rinse off with warm water.

SWEET AND GOOD YOGURT SCRUB

AD, PD, MD,
PCD

1 egg white   2 tablespoons brown sugar
½ cup yogurt

Beat egg white in a glass bowl until frothy. Add yogurt and sugar to egg white and carefully mix together. Gently rub your clean face with the mixture and rinse off with warm water.

OATMEAL AND HONEY SCRUB

1 tablespoon oats
1 tablespoon sunflower seeds

2 tablespoons yogurt
1 teaspoon honey, warm

A, P, M, C, PCA

In a blender, grind the oats with sunflower seeds. In a glass bowl, combine mixture with yogurt and honey. Gently massage onto your face, neck, or chest. Leave on for three minutes and then rinse off with warm water.

AVOCADO SCRUB

½ avocado
1 tablespoon cornmeal

1 teaspoon honey

AD, PD, MD,
CC, CD, PCC,
PCD

Mix all ingredients in a glass bowl. Dampen your face with warm water and gently massage in the scrub. Rinse off with warm water.

CREAM AND ALMOND SCRUB

1 tablespoon oats
¼ cup heavy cream

1 tablespoon almond meal
½ teaspoon honey

AC, AD, PC, PD,
MC, MD, CC,
CD, PCC, PCD

Use a blender to grind the oats. Mix all ingredients to form a creamy paste. (If it is too thick, add more cream. If it is too thin, add more oatmeal.) Gently massage the scrub onto your damp face, neck, and chest. Leave on for three minutes, then rinse off with warm water.

OLIVE OIL SCRUB

2 tablespoons almond meal
2 teaspoons olive oil

1 teaspoon grapefruit juice

AO, PO, MO,
CO, PCO

Combine all ingredients in a small bowl. Mix well and gently massage onto your face. Rinse off with warm water.

Masks

When applying a mask, always wash your face first and avoid the eye area. You can use a mask after a scrub.

JUST HONEY MASK

This takes advantage of honey's natural antibiotic properties.

A, P, M, C, PCA

2 teaspoons organic honey

Apply honey to your damp face and leave on for about fifteen minutes. Gently wipe off with damp flannel or a soft washcloth. You may use this mask up to three times a week.

EGG WHITE AND OATMEAL MASK

AO, PO, MO, CO, PCO

1 egg white
½ teaspoon lemon juice

⅓ cup cooked and cooled oatmeal (not instant)

Mix all ingredients in a bowl. Apply the mixture to clean, dry skin and leave on for twenty minutes. Gently wipe off the mask with tissues. Rinse your face with damp flannel or a soft washcloth.

CORNMEAL AND STRAWBERRY MASK

If you have a lot of inflammation, you can substitute peeled and crushed tomatoes for the strawberries.

AO, AC, PO, PC, MO, MC, CO, CC, PCO, PCC

⅓ cup cornmeal
4 or 5 strawberries (preferably organic), washed, hulled, and mashed

1 egg white
1 teaspoon New Zealand manuka honey
½ teaspoon lemon juice

Combine all ingredients into a paste. Apply to clean skin and leave on for ten to fifteen minutes. Rinse off the mask and follow with a hydrating gel, if needed.

AVOCADO REFRESHING AND SOOTHING MASK

AO, PO, MO, CO, PCO

½ avocado
1 tablespoon yogurt

1 egg white
⅓ teaspoon lemon juice

Mix all ingredients in a bowl. Apply to damp skin and leave on for ten to fifteen minutes. Rinse off with room-temperature water. Pat dry and follow with a non-comedogenic moisturizer.

Variation

½ avocado
1 tablespoon yogurt
½ teaspoon honey

½ teaspoon olive oil, coconut
  oil or almond oil

AD, PD, MD,
CD, PCD

Follow the same instructions as above.

TOMATO ON YOUR FACE

1 large tomato
1 teaspoon olive oil
½ teaspoon almond meal

1 teaspoon cornstarch
½ teaspoon rosemary leaves

AO, MO, PCO

Blend all ingredients to make a puree. Apply the mixture to clean, dry skin and leave on for fifteen minutes. Rinse off with warm water.

STRAWBERRY MASK

This mask can also be used on areas where you have breakouts.

1 egg white
3 or 4 large strawberries, hulled

1 tablespoon honey
1 tablespoon fine cornmeal

AO, PO, MO,
CO, PCO

Beat egg white in a glass bowl until frothy. Blend strawberries and honey. Add mixture and cornmeal to egg white and mix. Apply to a wet, clean face and leave on for twenty minutes. Rinse off with room-temperature water.

MILK MASK

2 tablespoons powdered milk
¼ cup yogurt

½ teaspoon honey

AD, PD, MC,
MD, CC, CD,
PCC, PCD

Mix all ingredients in a glass bowl until well blended. Apply to your face, neck, or chest. Leave on for fifteen minutes. Rinse off with room-temperature water.

OATMEAL WITH APPLES MASK

⅓ cup cooked oatmeal (not instant)
3 tablespoons applesauce

1 teaspoon vitamin E oil
1 tablespoon almond meal

A, P, C, PCA

Combine all ingredients in a glass bowl and mix well. Apply to your face, neck, or chest. Leave on for fifteen minutes. Rinse off with warm water.

BLUEBERRY MASK

A, P, M, C, PCA

⅓ cup blueberries
2 tablespoons yogurt

1 tablespoon rice flour

Place the blueberries in a glass bowl and smash them with a fork. Add other ingredients and mix well. Spread on your face, neck, or chest. Leave on for fifteen to twenty minutes. Rinse off with warm water.

Face, Neck, and Chest Moisturizers

These simple recipes use natural ingredients to hydrate, soothe, and deliver antioxidants as they moisturize your skin. For each recipe, simply mix all ingredients in a glass bowl and store in a sealed jar.

COCONUT AND ROSEMARY CREAM

AD, PD, MD, CD, PCD

½ cup base lotion
1 tablespoon coconut oil

1 teaspoon avocado oil
10 drops rosehip oil

CALENDULA AND CHAMOMILE CREAM

A, P, M, C, PCA

½ cup base cream
1 tablespoon almond oil
1 teaspoon calendula extract

5 drops calendula oil
5 drops chamomile oil

GREEN TEA MOISTURIZER

AO, PO, MO, CO, PCO

½ cup oil-free base lotion

1 teaspoon green tea extract

Variation

AC, AD, PC, PD, MC, MD, CC, CD, PCC, PCD

½ cup base cream

1 teaspoon green tea extract

CUCUMBER MOISTURIZER

½ cup oil-free base lotion
1 tablespoon cucumber extract

1 teaspoon chamomile extract
5 drops vitamin E oil

AO, PO, MO,
CO, PCO

Variation

½ cup base cream
1 tablespoon cucumber extract

1 teaspoon chamomile extract
5 drops vitamin E oil

AC, AD, PC, PD,
MC, MD, CC,
CD, PCC, PCD

THYME AND LEMON MOISTURIZER

½ cup oil-free base lotion
8 drops thyme oil
5 drops lemon oil

5 drops rosemary oil
8 drops calendula or
    chamomile oil

AO, MO, CO,
PCO

Eye Treatments

SOOTHING CUCUMBER GEL

½ organic cucumber, peeled
2 tablespoons aloe vera gel,
    refrigerated
½ tablespoon almond meal

2 small cotton pouches (these
    can be made from two circles,
    about the size of a CD, cut
    from a soft cotton fabric)
12" string, cut in half

A, P, M, C, PCA

Puree cucumber in a blender. Mix with aloe vera gel and almond meal.
Dampen cotton pouches with cool water. Put half of the mixture in each
pouch and secure with string. Place pouches on your closed eyes for ten
minutes. Pouches can be reused and stored in the refrigerator for up to
three days.

JUST THE TEA

⅓ cup water

2 chamomile tea bags

A, P, M, C, PCA

Boil water and brew tea. Steep for ten minutes. Remove bags and let
them slightly cool before placing one on each eye for five minutes. Dip
bags back into tea and place on eyes for another five minutes.

POTATO COMPRESS

A, P, M, C, PCA

1 potato (organic, if possible)

Cool potato in the refrigerator for one to two hours. Cut two ½-inch-thick slices. Place a slice on each eye for ten minutes. Rinse off eye area with cool water.

EVENING EYE TREATMENT

M, PCA

½ teaspoon shea butter   2 drops rosehip oil
¼ teaspoon jojoba oil

Combine all ingredients in a small jar. Mix well. After cleansing your face in the evening, gently massage a small amount around your eyes. You can also use this around your mouth.

AVOCADO NIGHT
EYE TREATMENT

AD, PD, M, C, PCA

1 teaspoon avocado   ¼ teaspoon yogurt or cream
¼ teaspoon avocado oil

Mix all ingredients in a small bowl. After washing and drying your face, apply a small amount around the eyes. Gently massage into the skin. You don't need to rinse it off.

ALMOND AND ROSEHIP OIL
EYE TREATMENT

M, C, PCA

1 teaspoon almond oil   4 drops vitamin E oil
¼ teaspoon rosehip oil

Mix all ingredients in a small jar. Shake well. After washing and drying your face, apply a small drop of oil and spread around the eye area.

Hand and Foot Treatments

MINTY FOOTBATH

4 cups water
4 mint tea bags
Italian parsley, crushed

Mint leaves, crushed
1 teaspoon lemon juice
2 tablespoons Epsom salt

A, P, M, C, PCA

Boil water and brew mint tea along with parsley and mint leaves. Add other ingredients and let cool. Fill a bowl, pan, or tub with warm water to soak your feet and add mixture. Soak your feet for ten to fifteen minutes.

SEA SALT SOOTHING FOOTBATH

2 tablespoons sea salt
1 tablespoon dry lavender flowers
2 drops geranium oil

2 drops lavender oil
1 drop rosemary oil

A, P, M, C, PCA

Fill your container for foot soaking with warm water. Add salt. Make sure it's dissolved before adding dry lavender flowers and oils. Soak your feet for ten to fifteen minutes.

CALENDULA FOOTBATH

1 cup water
½ cup dry calendula flowers
2 tablespoons calendula extract

2 teaspoons honey
2 tablespoons powdered milk

A, P, M, C, PCA

Boil water, add calendula flowers, and steep for five minutes. Fill your foot-soaking container with warm water. Add the calendula flower tea and all other ingredients. Stir well. Soak your feet for twenty minutes. Rinse with warm water, dry your feet, and apply a soothing calendula foot cream.

EUCALYPTUS FOOT SOAK

3 tablespoons Epsom salt
3 eucalyptus tea bags

5 drops eucalyptus oil

A, M, C, PCA

Place salt on the bottom of your foot-soaking container and add warm water. Drop tea bags and oil into the water. Let it sit for a bit and then soak your feet for twenty minutes.

OATMEAL FOOT AND HAND SOAK

A, P, M, C, PCA

3 cups milk   4 cups oats
2 cups water   2 tablespoons honey

Add milk, water, and oats to a saucepan on the stove. Cook until the oats gets soft. Slowly add cooked oats and warm water simultaneously to your foot-soaking container. Add honey and stir. Soak your feet (or hands) for fifteen to twenty minutes.

NUTTY FOOT OIL

A, P, M, C, PCA

1 teaspoon avocado oil or olive oil   1 teaspoon jojoba oil
1 teaspoon sesame oil   4 drops clover oil

Mix all ingredients and massage them onto your feet. Put on cotton socks so that the oils continue to absorb.

REFRESHING MINT FOOT LOTION

A, P, M, C, PCA

½ cup basic moisturizing lotion   4 drops peppermint oil

In a jar, mix lotion and peppermint oil. Massage a thin layer onto your feet.

COMFREY HAND AND FOOT CREAM

A, P, M, C, PCA

½ cup basic cold cream   1 teaspoon avocado oil
1 tablespoon comfrey extract

In a jar, combine all ingredients. Stir until they are well-blended. Massage the mixture onto your damp hands and/or feet right after a foot soak or a shower.

DRY CUTICLE MASK

A, P, M, C, PCA

1 teaspoon almond oil   ¼ avocado
½ teaspoon honey

Mix all ingredients in a glass bowl. Massage the mixture onto your cuticles. Leave on for twenty minutes and then rinse off with warm water. Apply hand cream.

CUTICLE CREAM

1 teaspoon cocoa butter   ½ teaspoon almond oil
½ teaspoon sunflower oil

A, P, M, C, PCA

Mix all ingredients in a glass bowl. Massage the mixture onto your cuticles. Leave on for twenty minutes and then rinse off with warm water. Apply hand cream.

REJUVENATING HAND TREATMENT

½ teaspoon olive oil   1 tablespoon cocoa butter
5 drops rosehip oil   ⅓ teaspoon vitamin E oil

A, P, M, C, PCA

Mix all ingredients. Massage onto your hands and put on cotton gloves that you can wear all night while you're sleeping.

Bath Soaks and Scrubs

ORANGE PEEL BODY SCRUB

Wrap clean orange peels in gauze. Rub on your skin while showering.

A, P, M, C, PCA

COFFEE IN THE SHOWER

1 cup finely ground coffee   2 tablespoons honey
⅓ cup olive oil or sesame oil

A, P, M, C, PCA

Brew coffee and mix with olive oil and honey. Gently rub the mixture on your body while in the shower. Rinse off with warm water.

ALMOND GREEN TEA SCRUB

⅓ cup oats   3 tablespoons green tea powder
⅓ cup almond meal   4 tablespoons olive oil

A, P, M, C, PCA

Use a blender to grind the oats. Combine all ingredients in a glass bowl until they form a paste. Massage the paste onto damp skin. Rinse off with warm water.

SUGAR AND MILK SCRUB

A, P, M, C, PCA

1 cup brown sugar

⅓ cup avocado oil or olive oil

⅓ cup half-and-half or heavy cream

2 tablespoons honey

Combine all ingredients in a glass bowl and mix into a paste. Rub the paste over damp skin. Rinse with warm water.

SWEET OATMEAL SCRUB

A, P, M, C, PCA

1 cup oats

⅓ cup warm honey

⅓ cup olive oil

8 drops ginger oil

Use a blender to grind the oats. Combine all ingredients in a glass bowl. Massage onto damp skin. Rinse off with warm water.

MILK BATH

A, P, M, C, PCA

1 cup water

4 chamomile tea bags or ½ cup
dry chamomile flowers

1 cup powdered milk

2 tablespoons sunflower oil

Boil the water and add the chamomile tea bags or dry flowers. Brew for fifteen minutes. Add the powdered milk and oil to running bathwater, then add the chamomile tea. (Bathwater should never be extremely hot.)

SOOTHING OATMEAL BATH

A, P, M, C, PCA

2 cups oats

⅓ cup dry green tea leaves

1 (10" by 10") piece of cheesecloth

String

Use a blender to grind the oats. Put all ingredients in the middle of cheesecloth and secure with string. Place pouch under running water as you fill the tub. (Bathwater should never be extremely hot.) Relax in the tub for twenty minutes. Once the water starts to cool, you may add more warm water.

ANTIOXIDANT HERBAL BATH

½ cup green tea leaves or
    5 green tea bags
3 pomegranate tea bags
2 tablespoons mint leaves or
    2 mint tea bags
2 tablespoons dry chamomile
    or 2 chamomile tea bags

1 tablespoon gingerroot or
    2 ginger tea bags
2 teaspoons grape extract
1 (10" by 10") piece
    cheesecloth
String

A, P, M, C, PCA

Put all ingredients in the middle of cheesecloth and secure with string. Place pouch under hot running water in the tub. When the bathtub is one-third full, change the water temperature to warm. Before you get in the tub, make sure the water is not too hot. Soak for fifteen to twenty minutes.

WARM HONEY BATH

½ cup honey
1 cup powdered milk

½ cup heavy cream or half-and-half
1 tablespoon calendula extract

A, P, M, C, PCA

Warm honey in a small pot on the stove. In a glass bowl, combine warmed honey with powdered milk. Mix in the other ingredients, then add the mixture to warm running bath water. Soak for fifteen minutes. Rinse well with warm water.

CITRUS BATH

½ cup orange juice
⅓ cup grapefruit juice
⅓ cup lemon juice

3 tablespoons lime juice
⅓ cup honey powder

A, P, M, PCA

Combine freshly squeezed juices with honey powder. Add the mixture to the bathtub under running water. Soak for fifteen minutes. Rinse well with warm water.

RELAXATION BATH

½ cup dry lavender
1 (10" by 10") piece cheesecloth
5 drops eucalyptus oil

4 drops peppermint oil
⅓ cup mint leaves
String

A, M, PCA

Place dry lavender on the cheesecloth and add drops of oil. Gently crush mint leaves in your hands and place them on top. Tie cheesecloth with string and place pouch under warm running water in the bathtub. Soak for fifteen to twenty minutes. Once the water starts to cool, you may add more warm water. Rinse well with warm water.

ALOE VERA BATH

A, P, M, C, PCA

2 cups water
3 chamomile tea bags
3 green tea bags

2 jasmine tea bags
2 cranberry apple tea bags
1 cup aloe vera juice

Place all tea bags in boiled water. Brew for fifteen minutes. Combine aloe vera juice with brewed tea. Under warm running water, add the mixture to your bathtub. Soak for twenty minutes. Rinse well with warm water.

Body Lotions

CALENDULA LOTION

A, P, M, C, PCA

½ cup base cream
1 teaspoon calendula oil

1 teaspoon avocado oil

Mix all ingredients in a glass bowl. Apply to damp skin right after a bath or shower. Store in a sealed jar.

BUTTER FOR YOUR BODY

A, P, M, C, PCA

⅓ cup shea butter
1 tablespoon avocado oil

1 tablespoon coconut oil
5 drops calophyllum oil

Mix all ingredients in a glass bowl. Apply body butter in a thin layer after a bath or shower. Store in a sealed jar.

GRAPE SEED BODY LOTION

A, P, M, C, PCA

½ cup base cream
¼ cup grape seed oil

1 teaspoon vitamin E oil

Mix ingredients in a tall container. Apply a thin layer after a bath or shower. Store in a sealed jar.

ALOE VERA BODY GEL

½ cup aloe vera gel
2 tablespoons dry calendula
  flowers

2 tablespoons dry chamomile
  flowers
1 teaspoon green tea leaves

A, P, M, C, PCA

Mix all ingredients in an ovenproof glass or clay container. Warm on the stove at a low heat setting for a few minutes until very warm. Cool completely, then pour the mixture through a fine sieve into a bottle or a jar.

CHAMOMILE BODY OIL

½ cup jojoba oil
1 teaspoon comfrey oil

1 teaspoon chamomile oil
5 drops vitamin E oil

A, P, M, C, PCA

Combine ingredients in a container with a tight lid and shake vigorously. Apply after bath or shower. Store at room temperature.

COCOA AND COCONUT CREAM

½ cup cocoa butter
2 tablespoons coconut base oil

1 tablespoon pure calendula
  cream

A, P, M, C, PCA

Mix all ingredients in a small bowl. Apply after a bath or shower.

Three Product Ingredient Lists with Breakdowns

NeoStrata Ultra Moisturizing Face Cream PHA 10

Ingredients: Aqua (water), gluconolactone, butylene glycol, isocetyl stearate, glyceryl stearate, PEG-100 stearate, cyclomethicone, isododecane, triethanolamine, palmitic acid, stearic acid, dimethicone, C12–15 alkyl benzoate, cetyl ricinoleate, *Macadamia ternifolia* seed oil, glycerin, cetearyl alcohol, diiostearyl malate, arginine, *Oenothera biennis* (evening primrose) oil, tocopheryl (vitamin E) acetate, magnesium aluminum silicate, steareth-2, xanthan gum, myristic acid, disodium EDTA, methylparaben, chlorphenesin, propylparaben.

The Top Third

1. **Aqua (water)**
2. **Gluconolactone** A polyhydroxy acid with antioxidant properties that is found naturally in fruit juice, wine, and honey; shown to protect from UV radiation and reverse signs of photoaging (pigmentation, wrinkling, enlarged pores); chelates (filters) metals and hydrates skin; gentle enough for use on sensitive skin or skin with rosacea.
3. **Butylene glycol** An alcohol used as a thinning agent, with some ability to add moisture; a common ingredient in skin care products for its gentleness even when used in high concentrations.
4. **Isocetyl stearate** Obtained from alcohol and animal or vegetable fats; serves as an emollient, a lubricant, and a degreaser and adds a thin hydrating film.
5. **Glyceryl stearate** A fatty acid naturally derived from soy or palm oil and used as a lubricant, an antioxidant, and a degreaser; forms a protective barrier to prevent moisture loss.
6. **PEG-100 stearate** A formulation of polyethylene glycol and a common ingredient in skin care products because of its emollient and emulsifying properties; controversial because of the risk of toxicity at high concentrations; should not be used on damaged skin.
7. **Cyclomethicone** A synthetic silicone oil that adds a slippery but nongreasy feel to products, adds surface moisture to the skin, and temporarily plumps fine wrinkles; does not penetrate the skin, so effects are not lasting.
8. **Isododecane** A petrochemical derivative that serves as an emollient and a fragrance carrier.
9. **Triethanolamine** Also known as TEA; derived from ammonia and ethylene oxide; used as a pH balancer, a buffering agent, and an emulsifier.

The Middle Third

10. **Palmitic acid** A saturated fatty acid derived from palm oil and other plant and animal sources; used as an emulsifier and a cleansing agent; can produce foam and may be drying.
11. **Stearic acid** A fatty acid derived from plant or animal sources; used as an emulsifier.
12. **Dimethicone** A commonly used synthetic silicone that forms a moisture-retaining barrier, adds a silky feel, and temporarily plumps fine lines.

13. **C12–15 alkyl benzoate**   A thickening and binding agent; forms a film that creates a silky touch; also used as a preservative for its antimicrobial effects.

14. **Cetyl ricinoleate**   A fatty acid derived from the oil of the castor bean and used as a non-comedogenic emollient and stabilizer; despite its name, this ingredient is not related to ricin, a poison derived from castor plants, and it has been approved for topical use by the FDA.

15. *Macadamia ternifolia* **seed oil**   The botanical source of the omega-7 palmitoleic acid; used as a moisturizer and an antioxidant; may trigger nut allergies.

16. **Glycerin**   A naturally occurring or synthetic ingredient that moisturizes and smoothes skin by balancing water levels; also contributes to effective skin-cell growth and turnover.

17. **Cetearyl alcohol**   A fatty alcohol, synthetic or derived from coconut oil; serves as an emulsifying wax, an emollient, a stabilizer, and a carrier of other ingredients.

18. **Diisostearyl malate**   An ester of fatty acids used as an emollient and a gloss; may cause dermatitis in sensitive skin.

The Bottom Third

19. **Arginine**   An essential amino acid that, in the body, helps stimulate blood flow and aid cell repair. Topically, it is used as an antioxidant and to hydrate and rebuild collagen.

20. *Oenothera biennis* **(evening primrose) oil**   The botanical source of gamma-linoletic acid, an omega-7 fatty acid; traditionally used in Chinese medicine as a skin soother and wound healer.

21. **Tocopheryl (vitamin E) acetate**   A fat-soluble form of vitamin E derived from plant, dairy, or animal sources; a natural antioxidant and moisturizer, but less acidic than pure vitamin E (tocopherol).

22. **Magnesium aluminum silicate**   A mineral derived from clay and used as a thickener; aluminum compounds have been associated with nerve damage, but this molecule is too large to penetrate skin and poses no risk in low concentrations.

23. **Steareth-2**   An emulsifier derived from propylene glycol and stearic acid.

24. **Xanthan gum**   Derived from glucose or sucrose; used as a stabilizer and a thickener; improves product shelf life.

25. **Myristic acid**   Also known as tetradecanoic acid; a fatty acid found in butterfat, nutmeg, coconut oil, and palm oil; used as an emulsifier, a cleansing agent, and a fragrance component.

26. **Disodium EDTA**   A salt of editic acid, used in most skin care products for its preservative and stabilizing qualities; chelates metals from hard water and keeps them from being deposited on the skin, so it is frequently found in rinse-off cleansers.

27. **Methylparaben**   A commonly used preservative and antifungal ingredient; controversial because it has estrogen-like effects and should therefore be avoided by people with estrogen-sensitive tumors; may cause sensitivity when used on broken or inflamed skin.

28. **Chlorphenesin**   An organic compound used pharmaceutically as a muscle relaxant; used in topical preparations at low concentrations for its preservative and antimicrobial properties; not recommended for use by pregnant women or around small children.

29. **Propylparaben**   A commonly used preservative and antifungal ingredient; controversial because it has estrogen-like effects and should therefore be avoided by people with estrogen-sensitive tumors; may cause sensitivity when used on broken or inflamed skin.

AVA MD DNA Repair Formula Age-Defying Serum

Ingredients: Purified water, isononyl isononanoate, ethylhexyl isononanoate, glycerin, propanediol, lecithin, sodium hyaluronate, *Santalum album* (sandalwood) extract, *Arabidopsis thaliana* extract, *Evodia rutaecarpa* fruit extract, plankton extract, *Phellodendrum amurense* bark extract, *Hordeum distichon* (barley) extract, micrococcus lysate, butylated hydroxytoluene, butylene glycol, acrylates, C10–30 alkyl acrylate crosspolymer, phenoxyethanol, disodium EDTA, caprylyl glycol, carbomer, chlorphenesin, sodium hydroxide.

The Top Third

1. **Purified water**
2. **Isononyl isononanoate**   An emollient and a skin conditioner; may cause contact dermatitis in sensitive skin.
3. **Ethylhexyl isononanoate**   Derived synthetically from grains; used as a preservative alternative to parabens; may cause allergic dermatitis in sensitive skin.
4. **Glycerin**   A naturally occurring or synthetic ingredient that moisturizes and smoothes skin by balancing water levels; contributes to effective skin cell growth and turnover.
5. **Propanediol**   An alkylizing chemical that corrects the pH balance of the skin.
6. **Lecithin**   Derived from soybeans; acts as an emulsifier and a mild preservative.
7. **Sodium hyaluronate**   The salt form of hyaluronic acid, naturally available in the body and derived from yeasts for cosmetic use; small molecules penetrate the skin for deep moisturizing and wrinkle reduction; an antioxidant that targets and corrects photodamage.
8. *Santalum album* **(sandalwood) extract**   A botanical oil derived from an Indian tree; a natural fragrance with anti-inflammatory properties.

The Middle Third

9. *Arabidopsis thaliana* **extract**   A botanical antioxidant extracted from mouse-ear cress plants.
10. *Evodia rutaecarpa* **fruit extract**   Also known as *wu zhu yu*, a botanical ingredient commonly used in Chinese medicine; has powerful anti-inflammatory properties when used topically.
11. **Plankton extract**   Derived from marine algae; adds moisture.
12. *Phellodendron amurense* **bark extract**   Also known as *huang bai*; a botanical derived from the cork tree, traditionally used in Chinese medicine for anti-inflammatory and antimicrobial properties; an alternative to parabens as a preservative.
13. *Hordeum distichon* **(barley) extract**   A botanical antioxidant that also serves as an emollient.
14. **Micrococcus lysate**   An enzyme derived from the micrococcus bacteria; recognizes and repairs UV damage to skin.
15. **Butylated hydroxytoluene**   Also known as BHT; a synthetic preservative used to prevent the oxidation of cosmetic ingredients; associated with health risks when taken internally, BHT is approved by the FDA for topical use only at very low concentrations.
16. **Butylene glycol**   An alcohol used as a thinning agent, with some ability to add moisture; a common ingredient in skin care products for its gentleness even when used in high concentrations.

The Bottom Third

17. **Acrylates**   Acrylic polymers used to stabilize ingredient blends, to create a waterproof seal, and as adhesives.
18. **C10–30 alkyl acrylate crosspolymer**   A thickening and binding agent that keeps ingredients from clumping; creates a film that seals in moisture.
19. **Phenoxyethanol**   Also known as ethylene glycol monophenyl ether; an antiseptic used as a preservative; may cause irritation and blistering.
20. **Disodium EDTA**   A salt of editic acid, used in most skin care products for its preservative and stabilizing qualities; chelates metals from hard water and keeps them from being deposited on the skin, so it is frequently found in rinse-off cleansers.
21. **Caprylyl glycol**   A plant-derived or synthetic alcohol that stabilizes and preserves ingredients; a moisturizer and an emollient.
22. **Carbomer**   A synthetic polymer that binds oils and water together, especially in gel products; can hold up to a thousand times its volume of water.
23. **Chlorphenesin**   An organic compound used pharmaceutically as a muscle relaxant; used in topical preparations at low concentrations for

THREE PRODUCT INGREDIENT LISTS WITH BREAKDOWNS 299

its preservative and antimicrobial properties; not recommended for use by pregnant women or around small children.

24. **Sodium hydroxide**   Also known as lye; used in low concentrations as a buffering agent and pH corrector.

Shikai All Natural Hand and Body Lotion—Pomegranate

Ingredients: Purified water, aloe vera (*Aloe barbadensis*) gel (certified organic), vegetable emulsifying wax, glyceryl stearate, apricot (*Prunus armeniaca*) kernel oil, avocado (*Persea grattissima*) oil, safflower (*Carthamus tinctorius*) seed oil, wheat germ (*Triticulum vulgare*) oil, glycerin, borage (*Borago officinalis*) seed oil, shea (*Butyrospermum parkii* fruit) butter, cocoa (*Theobroma cacao* seed) butter, dimethicone, cetyl alcohol, vitamin E acetate, ethylhexyl glycerin, natural fragrance, phenoxyethanol

The Top Third

1. **Purified water**
2. **Aloe vera (*Aloe barbadensis*) gel**   A botanical anti-irritant; promotes wound healing; used as a water-binding agent; certified organic
3. **Vegetable emulsifying wax**   A blend of the synthesized emulsifiers cetearyl alcohol, polysorbate 60, PEG-150 stearate, and steareth-20.
4. **Glyceryl stearate**   A fatty acid naturally derived from soy or palm oil and used as a lubricant, an antioxidant, and a degreaser; forms a protective barrier to prevent moisture loss.
5. **Apricot (*Prunus armeniaca*) kernel oil**   A botanical moisturizer and emollient.
6. **Avocado (*Persea grattissima*) oil**   A natural moisturizer and antioxidant.

The Middle Third

7. **Safflower (*Carthamus tinctorius*) seed oil**   A widely used botanical alternative to mineral oil; high in linoleic acid, a natural moisturizer.
8. **Wheat germ (*Triticulum vulgare*) oil**   A botanical antioxidant and moisturizer rich in vitamins, particularly vitamin E, and essential fatty acids; should be avoided by people with gluten allergies.

9. **Glycerin**   A naturally occurring or synthetic ingredient that moisturizes and smoothes skin by balancing water levels; contributes to effective skin-cell growth and turnover.
10. **Borage (*Borago officinalis*) seed oil**   A botanical source of gamma-linolenic acid (essential omega-6 fatty acid not found in the body but obtained through food); has proven anti-inflammatory and soothing effects.
11. **Shea (*Butyrospermum parkii* fruit) butter**   A botanical moisturizer, emollient, and antioxidant, with lipids that most closely match the skin's Natural Moisturizing Factor and oils produced by the sebaceous glands; seals in moisture, protects from irritation and infection; improves the appearance of dry, flaky skin; may trigger nut allergies.
12. **Cocoa (*Theobroma cacao* seed) butter**   A botanical fat used cosmetically as a skin softener; has natural preservative and fragrance properties.

The Bottom Third

13. **Dimethicone**   A commonly used synthetic silicone that forms a moisture-retaining barrier, adds a silky feel, and temporarily plumps fine lines.
14. **Cetyl alcohol**   A fatty alcohol derived from palm oil or as a by-product of petroleum refining; binds oil and water; acts as a thickener and an emollient.
15. **Vitamin E acetate**   Also known as tocopheryl acetate; a fat-soluble form of vitamin E derived from plant or animal sources; a natural antioxidant and moisturizer, but less acidic than pure vitamin E (tocopherol).
16. **Ethylhexyl glycerin**   Derived synthetically from grains; used as a preservative alternative to parabens; may cause allergic dermatitis in sensitive skin.
17. **Natural fragrance**   Pomegranate is an antioxidant, but this product uses only the fragrance.
18. **Phenoxyethanol**   Also known as ethylene glycol monophenyl ether; an antiseptic used as a preservative; may cause irritation and blistering.

RESOURCES

Dr. Ava Shamban
www.healyourskinthebook.com
DrAvaShamban@avamd.com

AVA MD Medical and Cosmetic Dermatology, Santa Monica
2021 Santa Monica Boulevard
Santa Monica, CA 90404

AVA MD Medical and Cosmetic Dermatology, Beverly Hills
9915 S. Santa Monica Boulevard
Beverly Hills, CA 90212

AVA MD Skin Recovery Clinic, Santa Monica
2021 Santa Monica Boulevard
Santa Monica, CA 90404

AVA MD Skin Recovery Clinic, Beverly Hills
9915 S. Santa Monica Boulevard
Beverly Hills, CA 90212

Cancer Support Community-Benjamin Center
1990 S. Bundy Drive, Suite 100
Los Angeles, CA 90025
310-314-2555
www.cancersupportcommunitybenjamincenter.org

Links to skin care products
http://www.lindiskin.com/
http://www.aveneusa.com/

INDEX